# BOOST
# YOUR BRAIN

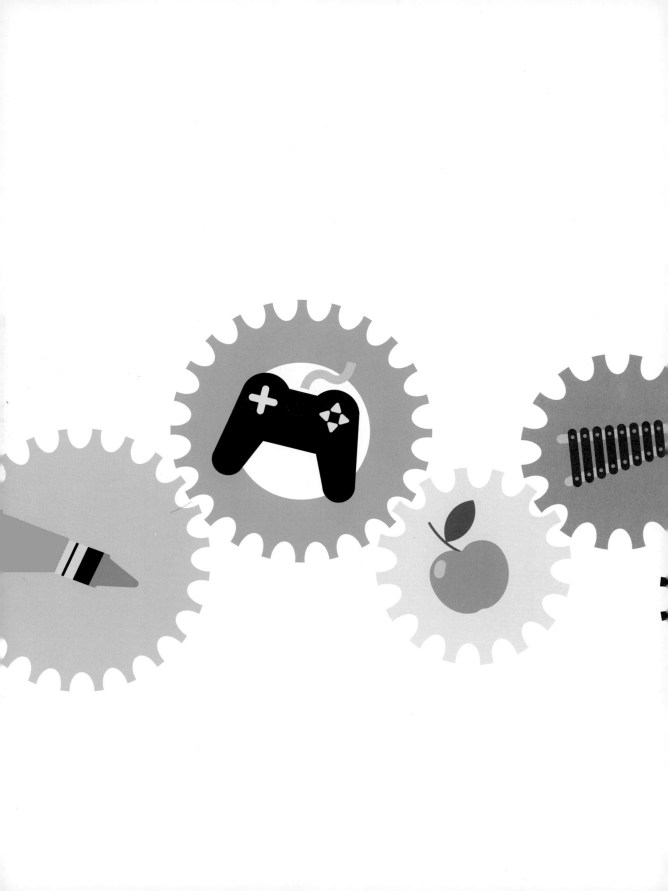

# BOOST
# YOUR BRAIN

## JOEL LEVY

**DK**

LONDON, NEW YORK, MELBOURNE,
MUNICH, AND DELHI

**Illustrator** Keith Hagan
**Project editor** Elizabeth Yeates
**Senior designer** Miranda Harvey
**Editor** Angela Baynham
**Designer** Harriet Yeomans
**Senior pre producer** Tony Phipps
**Senior producer** Jen Scothern
**Creative technical support** Sonia Charbonnier
**Managing editor** Dawn Henderson
**Managing art editor** Christine Keilty
**Art director** Peter Luff
**Publisher** Peggy Vance

First published in Great Britain in 2014
by Dorling Kindersley Limited
80 Strand, London WC2R 0RL Penguin Group (UK)

Copyright © 2014 Dorling Kindersley Limited

6 7 8 9 10
013–186655–Jan/2014

A CIP catalogue record for this book is available
from the British Library

ISBN 978-1-4093-2486-7

Printed and bound in China

**Discover more at
www.dk.com**

# Contents

HOW TO USE THIS BOOK 6
INTRODUCTION 8

## CHAPTER 1

QUICK FIX 10
**Short-term memory-boosting techniques
and exercises**
Questionnaire 12
Tip 21
Technique: chunking 22
Technique: associations 27

## CHAPTER 2

DINNER PARTY GENIUS 28
**Techniques and exercises for recalling
names and faces**
Questionnaire 30
Tip 31
Technique: names by location 32
Technique: what's in a name? 35
Technique: make it memorable 36
Technique: context is key 39
Technique: three-step booster 40

## CHAPTER 3

EVERYDAY ELEPHANT 42
**Developing techniques and exercises
for everyday challenges**
Questionnaire 44
Technique: memory house system 45
Technique: link system 46
Technique: acrostics tactics 48
Technique: alphabet peg system 50
Technique: rhyming number pegs 52
Tip 57

## CHAPTER 4

WHERE'S MY CAR?     58
**Medium-term memory-boosting techniques
and exercises**
Questionnaire     60
Technique: journey method     62
Technique: days of the week peg system     64
Tip     64
Technique: clock peg system     66

## CHAPTER 5

I KNOW WHAT I DID
LAST SUMMER     70
**Long-term memory techniques and exercises**
Questionnaire     72
Technique: explore the senses     74
Technique: cast list     75
Technique: calendar peg system     76
Tip     76

## CHAPTER 6

PIN IN A HAYSTACK     82
**Strategies for creating and remembering
PINs and passwords**
Questionnaire     84
Tip     85
Tip     91

## CHAPTER 7

REVISION EXPRESS     96
**Techniques and exercises for boosting revision
and recalling of facts**
Questionnaire     98
Technique: mnemonic acrostic     100
Technique: backgound check     101
Technique: topline     102
Technique: mental mapping     103
Technique: associations     104
Tip     104
Technique: body peg system     105

## CHAPTER 8

A HEAD FOR FIGURES     108
**Basic numeracy exercises**
Questionnaire     110
Tip     119

## CHAPTER 9

THE FEAR OF ALL SUMS     120
**More advanced numeracy puzzles**
Questionnaire     122
Tip     123
Tip     129

## CHAPTER 10

TIP OF THE TONGUE     130
**Verbal intelligence exercises**
Questionnaire     132
Tip     138

## CHAPTER 11

LOST IN SPACE     140
**Visuo-spatial intelligence exercises**
Questionnaire     142
Tip     147

## CHAPTER 12

LOGIC JAM     152
**Logical reasoning exercises**
Questionnaire     154
Tip     165

## CHAPTER 13

SPARK OF GENIUS     168
**Creativity exercises**
Questionnaire     170
Tip     176

CHALLENGES     178
ANSWERS     180
INDEX     188
ACKNOWLEDGMENTS     192

# Introduction

Everday life can push your mental abilities to the limit, whether it's remembering yet another website password or recalling the names of the people you were briefly introduced to at a dinner party. This book offers an intensive programme to help you face such challenges head on, with exercises and puzzles designed to boost all areas of your mental performance. In addition, it provides techniques and tips to tackle cognitive conundrums, giving you the expertise and confidence you need to overcome life's intellectual obstacles.

Before beginning your mental workout, take a moment to look at how your brain works and get acquainted with some helpful jargon. In everyday life you call on a variety of mental skills, which can be divided into two main types: memory and cognition. Memory covers everything from juggling prices in your head when shopping to recalling facts you learned at school. Cognition is a technical term for thinking, and includes intelligence, problem solving, creativity, and language aptitude.

## MEMORY

Nobody really knows for sure precisely how memory works, but experiments have suggested a model that seems like an accurate description: the multi-store model. According to this there are different stages of memory. Information detected by your senses floods into your brain and is held for only a second in a sensory register. Automatic filtering processes then let some of this information through into your short-term memory, which is sometimes known as working memory.

Only a few items of information can be held at a time in your short-term memory, where they remain for approximately 30 seconds before being either lost rapidly to decay and/or interference, or refreshed and reinforced through attention and repetition. For example, when you need to remember a phone number long enough to dial it, it's short-term memory that you are using – it is unlikely that you would remember the number for a long period of time. If, however, the material is interesting, emotional, chimes with other memories already stored, or if you make a conscious effort to rehearse and learn it, the material can be laid down as long-term memory, where an unlimited amount of information can remain indefinitely. Knowing how to tie your shoelaces is an example of long-term memory – it is continually "stored" in your memory.

The laying down of long-term memory, is called encoding. For information to be encoded and stored into your long-term memory, it must first pass through short-term memory. When encoded, memories are stored until you need to access them through the process known as recall. Encoding and recall are the two sides of the memory coin – unless you are able to do both of them, you won't remember something.

It is worth identifying an intermediate category, medium-term memory, which covers the area where short-term shades into long-term memory. Here, material can remain for approximately a week; it is the information that is not processed immediately from short-term to long-term memory, but will eventually either be stored in your long-term memory (through encoding) or will decay and be lost.

Long-term memory itself comes in several varieties. For instance, knowledge of skills, from driving a car to

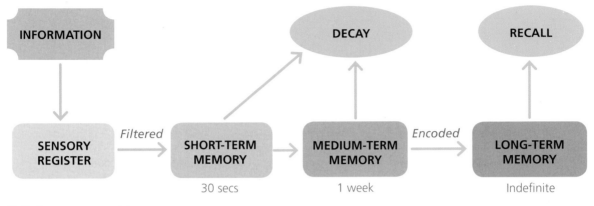

Multi-store memory model

typing to doing up your shoelaces, is called procedural memory – the "how" rather than "what". Memory for "what", such as "what year did the First World War begin?", is called declarative or explicit memory, and this itself breaks down into several forms. Episodic memory, for instance, is your memory for episodes and events in your life – events that have happened to you – and this includes a particular subset of episodic memory known as biographical memory. Biographical memory holds all your memorable personal experiences and is one of the most important forms of memory, as it is crucial to our sense of self.

Many problems and frustrations in everyday life are linked to poor or underperforming memory – from struggling to get into your online accounts to forgetting the one shopping item you went out for. Practising ways to improve each stage of memory formation and retrieval can improve mental performance in the short and long term; it may even help to counteract age-related memory decline.

## COGNITION

If memories are like the ingredients you store in your mental "larder", cognition is your ability to cook with them. Just as you might be good at chopping vegetables or an expert at baking, but hopeless at carving a roast or seasoning a sauce, the same applies to your mental processing, which breaks down into several subtypes or aptitudes. You may be more proficient in one area of cognition, and may need a little more practice in another.

Verbal, or linguistic, aptitude is your ability with words and language, which enables you to complete crosswords and determines whether you can turn a phrase or spell a tricky word. Numerical aptitude, is probably the area that elicits the most negative reactions, thanks to what is known as maths phobia.

Visuo-spatial aptitude covers your ability to think about shape, form, and space, and to represent physical space in your mind's eye. It determines how good you are at reading maps and finding your way, or holding a shape in your mind and then moving it around.

Logical aptitude is your ability to think rationally and solve puzzles, whether they involve words, numbers, or symbols. It underlies your ability to crack codes and solve puzzles such as Sudoku. Finally, creativity is an aspect of intelligence that covers your ability to make new and unexpected connections between ideas and be original and flexible in your thinking.

This is not the complete picture of intelligence; there is a whole other side to intelligence called emotional or social intelligence, which concerns your ability to recognize, control, and deal with your emotions and those of others. However, emotional intelligence is much more subjective and personal than rational intelligence, and doesn't lend itself to exercises and puzzles.

## JUMP TO IT

So, that's enough theory. Take a look at the pages on "How to use this book" then start at Chapter 1 (or the chapter most relevant to you) and enjoy boosting your brain!

# How to use this book

*Boost Your Brain* specifically addresses the mental challenges of modern living, with short digestible chapters that focus on a specific area, such as improving memory for passwords and PINs or tackling short-term forgetfulness "where did I put my keys?". Complete the exercises and learn memory-enhancing and brain-boosting techniques to give your brain a complete mental workout. Then discover how well you've performed and how you can improve.

## WORKING THROUGH THE BOOK

The book is divided into 13 chapters, each focusing on areas concerned with mental-agility challenges that can occur in everyday life, such as PINs, passwords, appointments, directions, and many more. You can turn straight to the chapter and area you feel you need to work on most, or proceed through the book systematically for an all-round mental fitness programme.

The first seven chapters focus on memory; Chapters 1–3 on short-term memory, Chapter 4 on medium-term memory, and Chapters 5–7 on long-term memory. Each of these chapters is task-orientated to maximize practical impact. For instance, Chapter 2 focuses on the problem of forgetting new names and faces, Chapter 6 targets the problem posed by the plethora of passwords and PINs people need to remember, and Chapter 7 explains techniques that can help improve your revision.

The remaining chapters deal with specific sub-types of intelligence. Chapters 8 and 9 deal with numerical intelligence, Chapter 10 with verbal intelligence, and Chapter 11 with visuo-spatial intelligence. Chapter 12 deals with logical reasoning, including riddles and codebreaking, while Chapter 13 focuses on creativity and lateral thinking.

Each chapter begins with a quick quiz to allow you to assess your capability in that particular field. You then dive straight into the exercises, puzzles, tips, and techniques.

Apart from Chapter 13, each chapter has a scoring system, which allows you to assess whether your brain is the best it can be or whether you need more practice. For Chapter 13, assess your own creativity by referring back to the exercises. Did you feel challenged by the activity? What would you do differently with hindsight?

A stopwatch symbol means there is a time limit on the exercise.

Brain-boosting technique boxes appear throughout the memory chapters and can help boost memory in everyday challenges.

Tip boxes offer helpful pointers that can boost performance in a chapter.

A scoring system determines how well you have performed in each chapter and gives advice on what to do next.

## TECHNIQUES AND TIPS

In the memory chapters, you will find in-depth explanations of memory-enhancing techniques and devices, known as mnemonics. These are strategies that top memory experts use to perform amazing feats of recall. These may seem challenging at first, but keep practising and they will become second nature, providing you with a powerful memory tool that you can use in many different aspects of daily life. Each chapter also has a tip box, offering quick tips to boost performance.

## TIMED TASKS AND BREAKS

Many of the exercises are time-limited to mimic "real-life" conditions, and these are indicated by a stopwatch symbol. In addition, many of the memory exercises suggest "time-lag" tasks, such as thinking of eight types of flower, for you to do between committing something to memory (encoding) and testing for recall. These time lags prevent you from mentally rehearsing the test material between encoding and recall by forcing you to focus on something else. You don't have to do the time lag task if you don't want to; you can just wait for a few minutes or create your own time lag, by making a cup of tea for example.

## SOLUTIONS

You will find the answers to the exercises for Chapters 1 to 12 at the back of the book (there's no scoring in Chapter 13). Add up your points and check the scoring system at the end of each chapter to see how well you performed. If you answered some of the exercises incorrectly, can you see where you went wrong? Look at the techniques and tips for guidance and try the exercises again. Even if you answered the exercises correctly, there is always room for improvement. See if you can challenge yourself further by solving the puzzles more quickly, or using the tips and techniques in your everyday life.

## CHALLENGES

Each chapter continues with a Challenge, which can be found at the back of the book. The Challenges are tasks to carry out at home, or during your daily routine. They are designed to lend a helping hand if your score in a chapter was disappointing, so that you can try to improve further in that area. Even if you scored well in a particular chapter, the Challenges are worth trying, as they can help to hone and maintain your mental abilities. The best way to keep your mind in tiptop condition is to keep using it, so keep referring to the Challenges to boost your brain beyond this book.

CHAPTER 1
# QUICK FIX
SHORT-TERM MEMORY

# Quick fix

Short-term memory (STM) is the human equivalent of RAM (random access memory) in a computer in that it is easy to manipulate and process, but also easy to erase and quick to fade. Is your short-term memory functional or failing?

## QUESTIONNAIRE
Use this quick quiz to get an instant rating of your STM skills.

**1** Do you ever walk into a room and then realize you've forgotten why you went into it?

Yes/No [score 1 point for "No"]

**2** When replying to questions by email, do you have to keep scrolling down the original email to see what the questions are?

Yes/No [score 1 point for "No"]

**3** You're on the phone and someone tells you a phone number; do you need to write it down straightaway, or can you wait until the phone call is over?

Write/Wait [score 1 point for "Wait"]

**4** You have called a taxi to come and pick you up from the airport. Can you remember the numberplate the firm gives you, so you can spot your waiting taxi among all the cars?

Yes/No [score 1 point for "Yes"]

**5** Stopping to ask for directions, you receive a list of six instructions. Will you have to stop and ask again before you reach your destination?

Yes/No [score 1 point for "No"]

**6** At the bar with six friends you take the drinks order. Do you need to write it down, or can you remember it all without help?

Write/Remember [score 1 point for "Remember"]

**How did you score?**
**0–2:** Your STM needs urgent attention. Give it a workout with the exercises in this chapter and check out the Challenge on page 178 for further development.

**3–4:** Your STM is average. Work on boosting it with this chapter's tests and quizzes.
**5–6:** Your STM is awesome! See if you can score top marks in the exercises that follow.

## 1 RANDOM OBJECT RECALL

Identify each of these objects and spell out the name of the object backwards. When you've done all eight, cover up the images and, using your STM, see if you can write down the whole list.

1 _____

2 _____

3 _____

4 _____

5 _____

6 _____

7 _____

8 _____

**8/8:** 1 point

**Your score** _____

## 2 WHERE DID YOU GET THAT HAT?

Can you spot the odd one out in this collection of hats? Once you've spotted it, cover up the pictures, then write down all the different types of hats your STM can recall.

1 _____

2 _____

3 _____

4 _____

5 _____

6 _____

6/6: 1 point

**Answer on page 180**

**Your score** _____

13

## 3 THESE CARDS WILL SELF-DESTRUCT

529661

4810246

942077312

02985385

3826564902

You're at a conference for spies, and some delegates have given you their business cards with their unique spy codes. There's just one hitch: the cards self-destruct after 30 seconds. Can you remember the numbers on the cards? For each number, read it once, cover it up then write it down on a piece of paper.

**What was the longest number you got right?**
**10 digits:** 5 points
**9 digits:** 4 points
**8 digits:** 3 points
**7 digits:** 2 points
**6 digits:** 1 point
**Your score** _____

## 4 ZOO TIME

Below are nine very different types of animal. Look at them for 30 seconds, then cover them up and see if you can recall all nine.

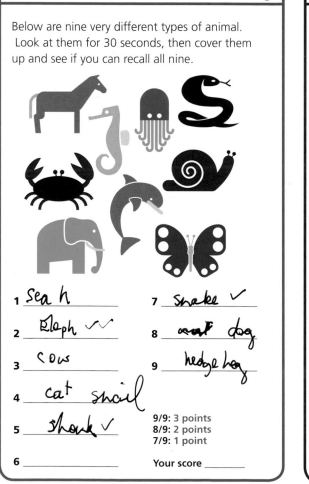

1  Sea h

2  Eleph ✓✓

3  Cow

4  cat  snail

5  shark ✓

6  _____

7  snake ✓

8  cat  dog

9  hedgehog

9/9: 3 points
8/9: 2 points
7/9: 1 point

**Your score** _____

## 5 BIRD TIME

Below are nine quite similar animals. Look at them for 30 seconds, then cover them up and see how your STM fares when you try to list all nine.

1  _____

2  _____

3  _____

4  _____

5  _____

6  _____

7  _____

8  _____

9  _____

9/9: 3 points
8/9: 2 points
7/9: 1 point

**Your score** _____

## 6 CAN YOU CUT IT?

Circle the items below that you would be able to cut with a knife.

**Answer on page 180**

Now cover the pictures and answer the questions below. Even though you weren't trying to memorize the objects, your STM has probably stored some of the details about them.

**What is on
top of the bun?** _____

**What is the logo on the
side of the kettle?** _____

**What colour is
the iron lead?** _____

**How many scoops of ice cream are there?**
_____

**Score 1 point for each correct answer**

**Your score** _____

## 7 AT THE SUPERMARKET

This exercise is another example of how your STM records information, such as locating and grouping, without you realizing. Which of these foods do you prefer to eat cooked, and which raw? Mark a "C" or an "R" above each item then cover the pictures.

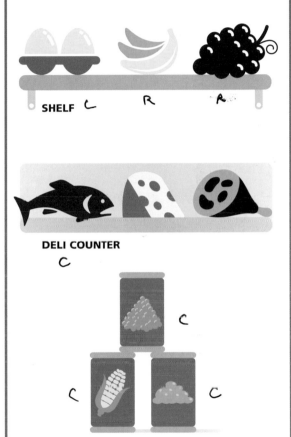

Can you remember which foods were where?

**Shelf** 1 _____ 2 _____ 3 _____

**Deli** 1 _____ 2 _____ 3 _____

**Tins** 1 _____ 2 _____ 3 _____

**Score 1 point for each trio of foods you got right**

**Your score** _____

# 8 BAR SIGNS

Here are eight bar signs. Study them for 5 seconds each, then cover them all and fill in the missing colours on the signs next door, writing the name of each bar below.

**8 names and colours/8:** 5 points  **7/8:** 4 points
**6/8:** 3 points  **5/8:** 2 points  **4/8:** 1 point

Your score _____

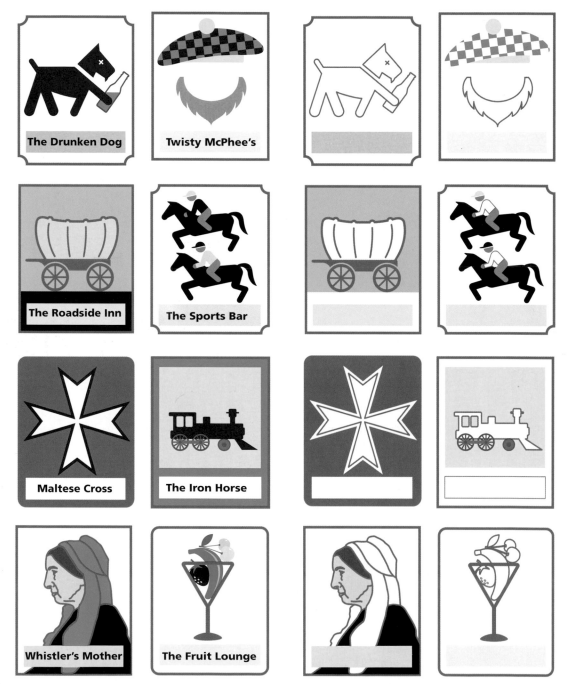

The Drunken Dog

Twisty McPhee's

The Roadside Inn

The Sports Bar

Maltese Cross

The Iron Horse

Whistler's Mother

The Fruit Lounge

# 9 TRAFFIC SIGNS

Traffic police are launching a crackdown on inattentive drivers who ignore the signs they see. Look through each sequence of signs separately for 10 seconds, cover it up, and fill in the blank below the sequence.

**Score 1 point for each correct answer**

**Your score** _____

**Dead end sign** was the _____ sign in the sequence

**Stop** was the _____ sign in the sequence

**Bear attack** was the _____ sign in the sequence

**Fork in the road** was the _____ sign in the sequence

# 10 DRAWING WITH YOUR MIND'S EYE

Can you draw a picture in your mind's eye and remember it for long enough to put it down on paper? Follow the instructions below in your head, cover the instructions, and draw what you can see in your mind's eye in the space provided.

Imagine a circle.
A square fits exactly inside the circle, touching the sides.
A diagonal line divides the square in half, running from top left to bottom right.
Sitting on top of the circle is a small triangle.
In the bottom left corner of the square is a black spot.

**Score 2 points** if your picture looks like the answer on page 180

**Your score** _____

## 11 DUCKS IN A ROW

You are stuck in a traffic jam caused by a line of seven unusual ducks crossing the road – see the seven ducks in the top row below. Now, cover them up and look at the seven ducks in the bottom row. Draw a circle around any duck in this row that was *not* crossing the road.

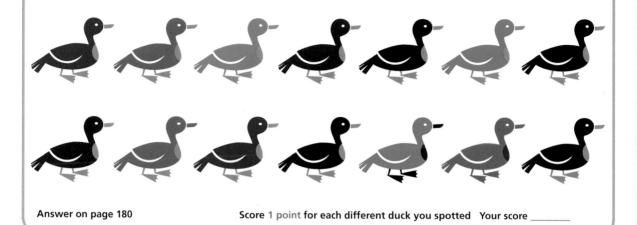

Answer on page 180

**Score 1 point** for each different duck you spotted   Your score _____

## 12 TRAIL BLAZER

You are leading a hike across dangerous country, but you manage only to glance at your map before a gust of wind blows it away. Look at the map on the left for 30 seconds, and then cover it up and fill in the appropriate landmarks on the blank map on the right.

**Score 1 point** for remembering all the landmarks   Your score _____

## 13 CHILD'S PLAY ⏱

Your toddler has been playing with the jewellery from a drawer in your jewellery box and has left 5 items on your bedside table. The first picture below shows how the drawer looked before she started playing with its contents. Look at this picture for 30 seconds, cover it up, and then draw arrows linking the items below the second picture to their rightful spots in the jewellery box.

**Score 1 point** for each piece of jewellery you put back in the right place

Your score _____

## 14 TREASURE ISLAND

A drunken pirate hands you a map of an island and gives you directions for finding treasure, before passing out. Read once through the directions below and then cover them up. Then trace a path across the map following the directions, starting from the spot marked "X".

**Directions:**

**A** Go north until you reach the third palm tree and then head west.

**B** Cross the swamp and the river to reach the cave.

**C** Head north across the mountains to the beach.

**D** Turn east and follow the river upstream to the third waterfall, then cross river.

**Where did you end up?** _____

**Answer on page 180**

**Score 2 points** for landing at the correct place

Your score _____

## 15 RACING COLOURS

There's panic at the Grand Prix as unusual weather conditions have resulted in mud all over the paintwork on the racing cars. Can you help restore their racing liveries by reading through the team colour descriptions in the programme (right), covering the descriptions, and then colouring in the cars below, one team at a time? If you don't have coloured pens or pencils handy, just write in the name of the colour.

**Team Boost:** Green front spoiler, blue nose, red cockpit, orange body, yellow rear spoiler

**Team Sprint:** Blue front spoiler, orange nose, yellow cockpit, blue body, green rear spoiler

**Team SuperX:** Red front spoiler, orange nose, green cockpit, yellow body, blue rear spoiler

**Team WarpSpeed:** Blue front spoiler, red nose, orange cockpit, green body, yellow rear spoiler

**Team Vanish:** Yellow front spoiler, orange nose, red cockpit, blue body, green rear spoiler

**Team Boost**          **Team Sprint**          **Team SuperX**          **Team WarpSpeed**          **Team Vanish**

**Score 1 point for each team livery you got completely right   Your score** _____

## 16 CONTEXT IS KING

**A** At a tennis match: the order of priorities for survival is shelter, water, food.

**B** On a bus: the scientific notation for the element gold is Au.

**C** In the rain: the capital of Uruguay is Montevideo.

The trouble with STM is that things can slip out of it as quickly as they go in. One way to fix things more firmly in your STM is to pay close attention to the context in which you receive information. Try this out by reading the three facts on the left in the context of the suggested scenario. You'll be tested on the information later in the chapter.

# 17 CHESS CHALLENGE

You are playing chess in the park, but the wind keeps blowing over the pieces. For each game below, look at the first board for 30 seconds, then cover it up and reproduce it on the empty board alongside.

**Score 2 points for each board you got right**

**Your score** _____

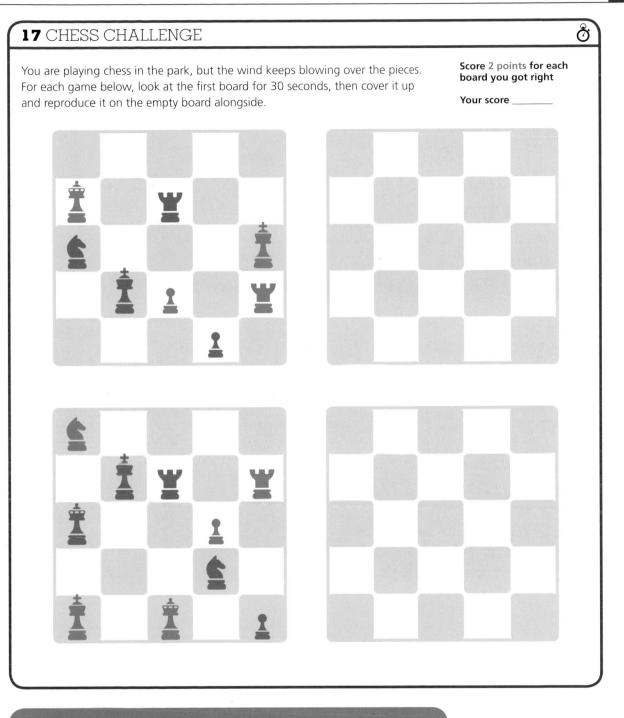

**TIP** STM by its nature fades very quickly. A simple tactic to counteract this is instant review, where you immediately repeat new information in your head or, even better, out loud.

## 18 KIM'S GAME

In Rudyard Kipling's 1901 novel *Kim,* part of a spy's education involves memory training. In this simple game, memorize the objects below for 30 seconds and then cover them up. On a separate piece of paper, list as many objects as you can.

**14–15: 3 points**
**12–13: 2 points**
**10–11: 1 point**

**Your score** _____

**TECHNIQUE: CHUNKING**

Chunking means organizing information into chunks. Your STM can handle only around seven pieces of information at a time, but if you can organize multiple bits into a single chunk, it may help you to cram more in. Try memorizing these 14 objects as seven pairs. Then cover them up, wait 30 seconds, and on a separate piece of paper, see if you can list them all.

## 19 KIM'S GAME: HARD

The objects below are more similar to each other than those In exercise 18 and therefore less memorable. Using chunking, pair up the items and see how many you can recall when you cover them up after 30 seconds of memorizing.

**14:** 5 points  **12–13:** 4 points
**10–11:** 3 points  **7–9:** 2 points
**6:** 1 point

**Your score** _____

## 20 KIM'S GAME: FIENDISH

Only memory champions will succeed in this tough challenge! Using chunking, give yourself 30 seconds to memorize these 30 items, then see how many of them you can write down on a piece of paper.

**25–30:** 10 points  **17–24:** 8 points
**12–16:** 6 points  **10–11:** 4 points
**8–9:** 3 points  **6–7:** 2 points  **5:** 1 point

**Your score** _____

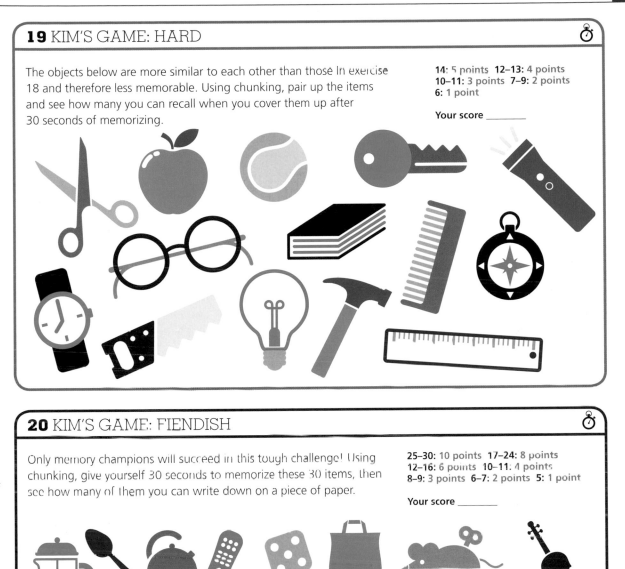

## 21 CONTEXT IS KING

**A** At a tennis match

**B** On a bus

**C** In the rain

Earlier in the chapter (exercise 16) you were given three bits of trivia to remember. With the contexts as cues, can you remember the information?

**Fact:** _____

**Fact:** _____

**Fact:** _____

**Score 1 point** for each fact you remembered

**Your score** _____

## 22 FADE AWAY

STM is especially vulnerable to "decay", where the information stored fades away and is forgotten. People with less decay have better memories. For a quick test of your decay rate, see if you can remember the answers to some of the previous questions:

**1. Name two of the types of hat from exercise number 2 "Where did you get that hat?"**

_____  _____

**2. Which hat was the odd one out in that exercise?** _____

**Score 1 point** for each correct answer

**Your score** _____

**3. Name four of the animals from exercise number 5 "Bird time".**

_____  _____

_____  _____

**4. From the technique on "Chunking", name one of the object pairs.** _____

**5. Name two of the objects from exercise number 18 "Kim's game".**

_____

_____

## 23 BACKGROUND NOISE

Keeping information in your STM becomes much harder when you are coping with distractions. Try this exercise, for instance: on the right is a hand of cards – can you memorize the hand in 30 seconds while counting backwards from 113 in multiples of 3 (i.e. 110, 107, 104, and so on)? When the time is up, cover the cards and write down the hand.

**5/5: 2 points  4/5: 1 point   Your score** _____

## 24 INTERFERING OBJECTS

Another problem with STM is called "interference". This is where new information coming in to your STM interferes with previous storage, causing you to forget it. How well can you cope with interference?

**A** Give yourself 30 seconds to memorize the set of objects below, then cover them up and move on to task B.

7/7: 3 points  5–6/7: 2 points  3–4/7: 1 point

Your score _____

**B** Draw a circle around which one of these is the odd one out.

**Answer on page 180**

**C** Can you remember the objects memorized in part A?

1 _____    5 _____

2 _____    6 _____

3 _____    7 _____

4 _____

## 25 INTERFERING NUMBERS

Try another exercise to see how well you can cope with interference.

**A** Memorize this sequence of numbers for 10 seconds, then cover them up: **4 2 9 0 6 4 8**

**B** What comes next in this series of playing cards?

_____

**Answer on page 180**

**C** What were the numbers you memorized? _____

7/7: 2 points  6/7: 1 point

Your score _____

## 26 NATURAL WONDERS

Retrieving things from your STM is much easier when you have a cue or trigger to help you remember the information. Allow 30 seconds to remember which natural wonder is in which country, then cover the list.

**Angel Falls:** Venezuela          **Mount Everest:** Nepal

**Table Mountain:** South Africa

**Great Barrier Reef:** Australia

**Blue Grotto:** Italy

**Kilimanjaro:** Tanzania

**Grand Canyon:** USA

Now using the list of countries below, write down the natural wonder associated with each.

**Australia:**_____

**Nepal:**_____

**Tanzania:**_____

**Italy:**_____

**USA:**_____

**South Africa:**_____

**Venezuela:** _____

Score 1 point for each correct answer

Your score _____

## 27 LOVE LINKS

Information with emotional content or associations is often easier to remember. Read through this list of relationships, then cover it all and answer the question.

Ben and Omar are old school friends.

Ted and Katie have been married for 40 years.

Dave is falling in love with Zoe.

John and Orla are having a baby together.

Jessica and Bill are getting divorced.

Karen and Dave are having an affair.

Winona and Desirée are identical twins.

**Which couple is having a baby?** _____

Score 1 point for a correct answer

Your score _____

**TECHNIQUE: ASSOCIATIONS**

Another way to fix new information more firmly in your STM is to build associations between it and information you already know, such as famous names and faces. For instance, try remembering a hand of cards by associating the individual cards with famous names. For example, study the cards below and the associated famous names for 30 seconds. Then cover the cards and spell out the titles of three of your favourite films. Can you remember the cards by thinking of their association?

**Brad Pitt    Angelina Jolie    Mark Zuckerberg    Bill Gates    Meryl Streep**

## 28 DRINKS ORDER

It's your turn to go to the bar, but you don't have a pen and paper to write down the drinks. To remember the order, associate each drink below with the face or name of the friend who ordered it. Can you remember who ordered which drink?

Charles wants **champagne**

Adam wants **martini**

Martin wants a **pint of beer**

Brenda wants a **glass of red wine**

Val wants a **pint of stout**

Don wants a **bottle of lager**

6/6: 3 points  5/6: 2 points
4/6: 1 point

Your score _____

Your score  /100

**80–100 GOLD**
Your STM is excellent, but to maintain and maximize high performance it may help to try the Challenge on page 178.

**30–79 SILVER**
Your STM could be improved. Go back and look at the tips for STM boosting, and check out the Challenge on page 178.

**0–29 BRONZE**
Your STM needs work. Try the exercises in the chapter again to help boost your performance.

Turn to page 178 for the Challenge.

CHAPTER 2
# DINNER PARTY GENIUS
NAMES AND FACES

# Dinner party genius

Humans have specialized brains and mental processes for perceiving and recognizing faces. Unfortunately, memory often lets us down – especially when we fail to transfer name–face associations from short-term to long-term memory.

## QUESTIONNAIRE
Use this quick quiz to get an instant rating of your memory for names and faces.

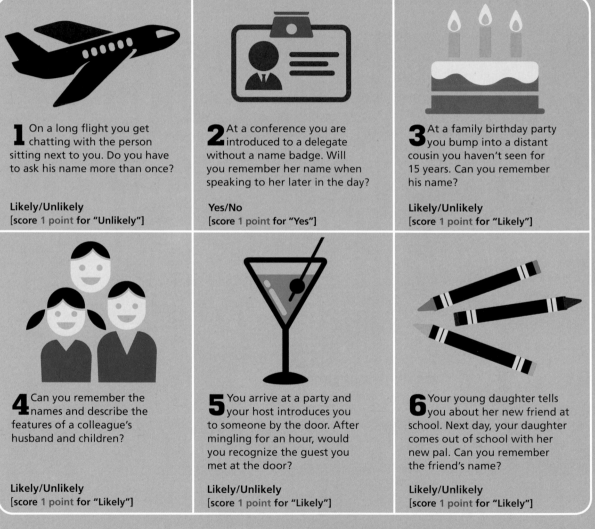

**1** On a long flight you get chatting with the person sitting next to you. Do you have to ask his name more than once?

**Likely/Unlikely**
[score **1 point** for "Unlikely"]

**2** At a conference you are introduced to a delegate without a name badge. Will you remember her name when speaking to her later in the day?

**Yes/No**
[score **1 point** for "Yes"]

**3** At a family birthday party you bump into a distant cousin you haven't seen for 15 years. Can you remember his name?

**Likely/Unlikely**
[score **1 point** for "Likely"]

**4** Can you remember the names and describe the features of a colleague's husband and children?

**Likely/Unlikely**
[score **1 point** for "Likely"]

**5** You arrive at a party and your host introduces you to someone by the door. After mingling for an hour, would you recognize the guest you met at the door?

**Likely/Unlikely**
[score **1 point** for "Likely"]

**6** Your young daughter tells you about her new friend at school. Next day, your daughter comes out of school with her new pal. Can you remember the friend's name?

**Likely/Unlikely**
[score **1 point** for "Likely"]

### How did you score?
**0–2:** Your memory for names and faces needs work, and may prove to be seriously embarrassing if not addressed. Work through the techniques and exercises in this chapter and see how you can improve it.

**3–4:** Your memory for names and faces is average. Use the techniques and exercises in this chapter to boost your performance.

**5–6:** Your memory for names and faces is impressive. Stretch yourself to the limit with the tests in this chapter.

## 1 FUNNY FACES

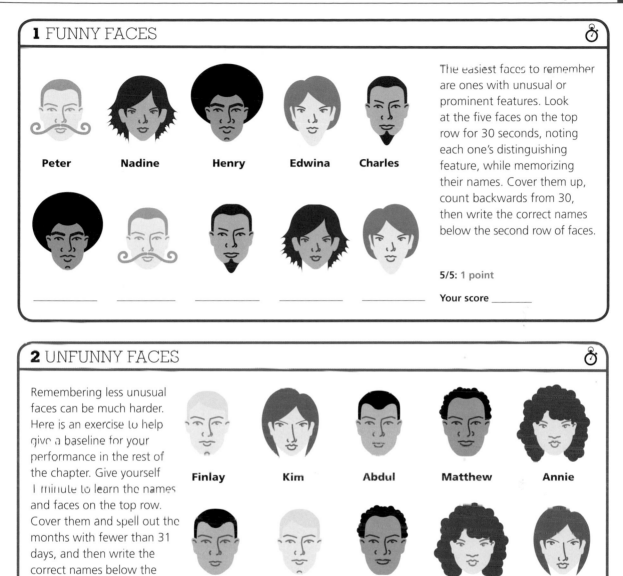

Peter    Nadine    Henry    Edwina    Charles

The easiest faces to remember are ones with unusual or prominent features. Look at the five faces on the top row for 30 seconds, noting each one's distinguishing feature, while memorizing their names. Cover them up, count backwards from 30, then write the correct names below the second row of faces.

5/5: 1 point

_____    _____    _____    _____    _____    **Your score** _____

## 2 UNFUNNY FACES

Remembering less unusual faces can be much harder. Here is an exercise to help give a baseline for your performance in the rest of the chapter. Give yourself 1 minute to learn the names and faces on the top row. Cover them and spell out the months with fewer than 31 days, and then write the correct names below the bottom row of faces.

Finlay    Kim    Abdul    Matthew    Annie

_____    _____    _____    _____    _____

5/5: 2 points 4/5: 1 point    **Your score** _____

**TIP**

The simplest way to boost your memory for names is to repeat the name as soon as you hear it. This will help imprint the name into your brain for future recall. Another good way to work in repetition when you first meet someone is to reframe your introduction as a question. For instance, you might say, "Arthur Deeley was it? Is that spelled DEELEY or DEALEY?" Practise doing this each time you are introduced to somebody new.

TECHNIQUE: NAMES BY LOCATION

It can be useful to visualize a plan of who is positioned where and to remember their names according to their location. Imagine you have flown with a tour party to Barcelona, Spain. On the return journey, the tourists sit in the same seats on the plane, but they no longer have name badges. Use their positions on the seating plan below to help you memorize names for 1 minute, then cover it up. Wait another minute, then answer the questions below.

| Row 1 | Row 2 | Row 3 | Row 4 |
|---|---|---|---|
| **A** Billy Chan | **A** John Marks | **A** Paul Alberts | **A** Harry James |
| **B** Louise Smith | **B** Jane Gregg | **B** Tony Graham | **B** Liz Adam |

**1** Who is in seat **2A**? _____

**2** Which seat is **Tony Graham** sitting in? _____

**3** Which two people are sitting in **Row 4**? _____

**4** Which seat is **Louise Smith** sitting in? _____

# **3** GUEST HOUSE GUESSER

You have arrived at a guest house for the weekend with friends of your partner. Can you remember who is with whom and in which room each couple is staying? Memorize the list of couples and in which room they are staying for 1 minute, then cover the list and fill in the couples' names in the boxes on the room plan (right).

John and Jill are in the **Master bedroom**

Barbara and Kenneth are in the **Snug**

Lucy and Gokwan are in the **Hearth room**

Robert and Pamela are in the **Gazebo room**

Score **1 point** for each couple placed correctly
Your score _____

## 4 DINNER PARTY CHALLENGE ⏱

You arrive late at a dinner party and your hostess makes a quick round of introductions. Study the list of names, faces, and seating positions below for 1 minute, then cover it up and take your seat at the table. Can you remember who is sitting where?

**Martha**, sitting on your right

**Leo**, sitting opposite you

**Jeff**, sitting on Leo's left

**Andrew**, sitting at the end nearest to you (on your left)

**Louise**, sitting at the far end of the table

YOU

**5 correct names/5: 1 point   Your score _____**

## 5 SCHOOL DAZE ⏱

It is your first day in a new class and the teacher asks you to distribute the papers he has just graded – but you've only had a short while to learn who is sitting where. Can you hand out the papers to the correct student? First study the seating plan below for 2 minutes, then cover it up and name 10 American states. Now write the names of the children in the blank spaces below.

| Sarah | Frank | Julie |
| Jamilla | Henry | James |
| George | Samantha | Lucinda |
| Gary | Edward | You |

1 _____  2 _____  3 _____

4 _____  5 _____  6 _____

7 _____  8 _____  9 _____

10 _____  11 _____  You

**11/11: 5 points  9–10/11: 4 points  7–8/11: 3 points**
**5–6/11: 2 points  3–4/11: 1 point   Your score _____**

33

## **6** ORDER ORDER

Recalling not just the names of people you have been introduced to but the order in which they were introduced might sound tricky, but if you can put the names into a simple but memorable narrative (a series of connected events), it could boost recall.

Try to think of a narrative sequence with the characters below. After 2 minutes, cover up the names and faces, then name five James Bond films. Write down the names beneath the bottom row of faces and give the position each appeared in the sequence.

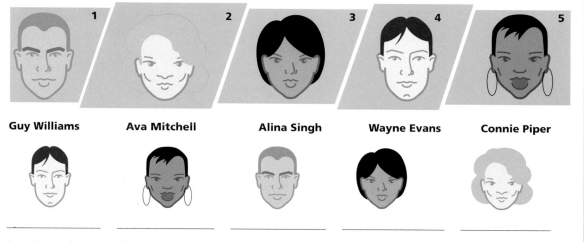

**Guy Williams**   **Ava Mitchell**   **Alina Singh**   **Wayne Evans**   **Connie Piper**

Score **1 point** for each full name, and another **1 point** if you listed all of them in the right order   Your score _____

## **7** NOMINATIVE DETERMINISM

When someone's job matches their name it is known as nominative determinism. It makes for a helpful mnemonic aid (a memory-enhancing technique). Memorize these names using their work association, cover, then list them:

1 _____

2 _____

3 _____

4 _____

5 _____

6 _____

7 _____

7/7: 1 point

Your score ____

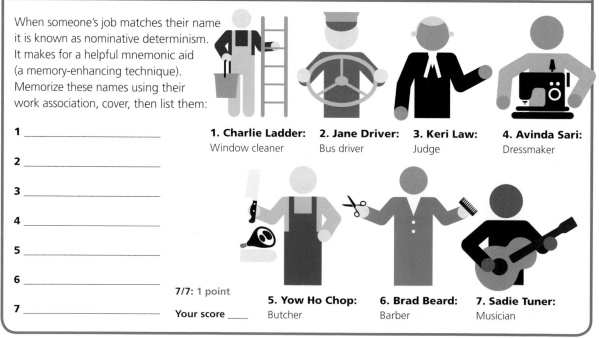

**1. Charlie Ladder:**
Window cleaner

**2. Jane Driver:**
Bus driver

**3. Keri Law:**
Judge

**4. Avinda Sari:**
Dressmaker

**5. Yow Ho Chop:**
Butcher

**6. Brad Beard:**
Barber

**7. Sadie Tuner:**
Musician

**TECHNIQUE: WHAT'S IN A NAME?**

People with names that immediately suggest a visualization or association are a gift to someone of poor memory. For each of these four people, think of an obvious visualization or association. For instance, you might remember Mr Butterman by visualizing him being spread on toast. Once you've got your memory cues for the other three names and faces, cover the names beneath the faces and see if you can use your visualizations to recall their names.

**Mr Butterman**     **Miss Plum**     **Mr Golightly**     **Mrs Atticus**

_____   _____   _____   _____

## 8 MEET THE INTERVIEW PANEL

You want to make a good impression at an interview, but everyone in the panel is dressed alike. Can you remember who is who? Using the technique above, try making a visualization or association with these less memorable names. Study the names above the panel for 30 seconds, then cover them up and recite every third letter of the alphabet. Now try to recall the names.

**Mr Poole**     **Ms Nolan**     **Mr Basu**     **Mr Goodall**     **Mrs Hall**

_____  _____  _____  _____  _____

**5/5: you're hired! 1 point   Your score** _____

**TECHNIQUE: MAKE IT MEMORABLE**

Boost memory by using correspondences between names and how a person looks. First, focus on an individual's features, then see if you can make a memorable visualization linking their features to their name. To practise this, give yourself 2 minutes to jot down on a separate piece of paper memorable visualizations linking each of these name/face combos. Then cover up the faces and your visualization, and see if you can recall the names.

**Tilly Flower**     **Duncan Large**     **Ernest Monkton**     **Pepper Prado**     **Sampson Ching**

# 9 TRAIN CHARACTERS

To practise this technique, begin by just remembering people according to their features. Six unusual-looking passengers share your train carriage on a long journey. The next day you try to describe to a friend what they all looked like. Study the passengers below left, then cover them up and wait 5 minutes. Now write down the missing distinguishing features for the faces on the right.

**Score 1 point for each correct feature   Your score _____**

## 10 IDENTIKIT

Now practise making associations between names and features with this exercise. Study the five pictures in the top row and memorize the features for each name, then cover them, name the titles of the last three books you read, then see if you can remember the name that goes with each face.

**Polly Turner**     **Sunil Batra**     **Joe Seymour**     **Augustine Brown**     **Jade Pike**

## 11 IF THE NAME FITS

Now combine names and features with a visualization. At Great Aunt Greta's 80th birthday party you can't remember the names of half your relatives. Your sister gives you a quick run down: give yourself 1 minute to connect these names and faces with visuals, then cover them up and, on the right, fill in the name below the relative, as well as drawing in their missing feature.

Score **1 point** for each correct name and **1 point** for each correct feature

Your score _____

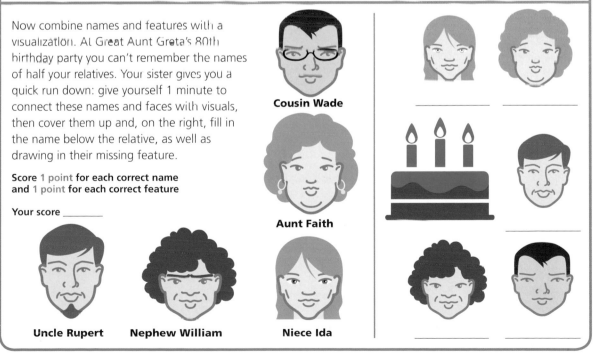

**Cousin Wade**

**Aunt Faith**

**Uncle Rupert**     **Nephew William**     **Niece Ida**

## 12 COUPLING UP

If you find it difficult remembering people's names, then recalling the names of their partner may be even harder. Try using some of the techniques you've learned to memorize who is with whom. Below are four couples. Use their names or memorable features as the basis for associations, then cover them up. Move on to exercise 13, then come back to fill in the blanks on the right.

Who is **Celeste** with? _____

is with _____

Who is **Abdul** with? _____

is with _____

Who is **Felix** with? _____

is with _____

**Harry and Meg**

**Celeste and Arthur**

**Abdul and Fatima**

**Ruby and Felix**

6/6: 1 point   Your score _____

## 13 WE COME IN PEACE

This extra-tough challenge requires you to remember alien appearances and names. Aliens have landed and selected you to be Intergalactic Ambassador for Humanity. It is essential you follow protocol and remember each alien's name. Study the aliens and their names below for 2 minutes, cover them, and name the last five films you have watched. Then connect the names to the aliens pictured below.

Score **1 point for each alien's name you correctly recalled**

Your score _____

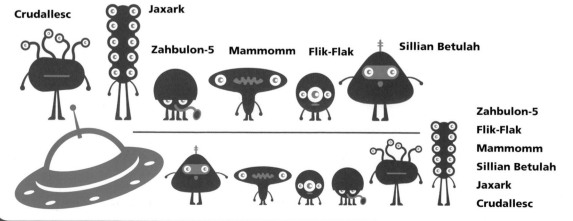

Crudallesc

Jaxark

Zahbulon-5   Mammomm   Flik-Flak

Sillian Betulah

**Zahbulon-5**

**Flik-Flak**

**Mammomm**

**Sillian Betulah**

**Jaxark**

**Crudallesc**

## TECHNIQUE: CONTEXT IS KEY

By giving context to any new introduction you can help boost your recall. Pay attention to the circumstances around an introduction – where you were, what was in the background, what was the occasion, and so on. Use these examples as practice. Give yourself 2 minutes to learn them, name 12 European countries, then see if you can remember who is who.

**Phillipa** you met on a windy day

**Vanessa** you met on a visit to London

**Ardal** you met at a firework display

**Imogen** was carrying roses when you met

**Nishit** you met on a plane

---

## 14 TESTING TIMES

Can you remember the names of these school teachers and their subjects? Study the list for 1 minute, using the topics of the lessons and the classroom setting to forge a memorable visualization with each teacher's name. Then cover it all, complete exercise 15, and come back and see if you can write their names and subject below.

1 _____

2 _____

3 _____

4 _____

5 _____

6 _____

Score 1 point for each correct name
Your score _____

**Mrs Proud (History)**

**Mr D'Angelo (Art)**

**Mr Edwards (Geography)**

**Ms Farnborough (Literature)**

**Mrs Hwan (Physics)**

**Mr Letterman (Biology)**

**TECHNIQUE: THREE-STEP BOOSTER**

Putting together some of the tips used in this chapter so far results in a technique called the three-step booster. This involves using a person's name to suggest one memorable association, using their facial features to suggest another association, and then combining the two to create an overall super-memorable association. In the example below, you can associate Linda Scott's name with a Scottie dog and her hair style with a beehive, then combine the two in a memorable image: the Scottie dog chasing bees. Can you do the same with David Hooper?

Linda Scott

David Hooper

**Name association**

Scottie dog

**Feature association**

beehive

**Link**

_____  _____

_____  _____

## **15** UNFORGETTABLE FACES

Use the three-step booster technique to memorize these four name–face combos. Think of an association for each name and then an association for each face, then link the two associations in a memorable image. Now cover the names, associations, and links and think of 12 types of birds. Then, on a separate piece of paper, see if you can write down the name that goes with each face.

| | | **Name association** | **Face association** | **Link** |
|---|---|---|---|---|
| | Chavez 1 | | | |
| | | | | |
| | Aminah 2 | | | |
| | | | | |
| | Fion 3 | | | |
| | | | | |
| | Fawcett 4 | | | |
| | | | | |

Score **1 point** for each name you remember   Your score _____

# 16 TRADE PLACES

You are sent to welcome a trading delegation from China, but your boss turns up and wants to be introduced to each person. You heard the guests' names only once and now you have to remember them or risk causing offence! Can you put your three-step booster technique to the ultimate test by rapidly forging robust visualizations after looking at the list of names and features only once? Cover the names and your links, name seven newspapers, and see if you can write down each guest's name on a separate piece of paper.

| | Name association | Face association | Link |
|---|---|---|---|
| **Wu Zhaoxu** 1 <br> Head of the delegation | | | |
| **Song Bingguo** 2 <br> Assistant to Mr Wu Zhaoxu | | | |
| **Gao Lei** 3 <br> Only woman in the delegation | | | |
| **Qin Lingyu** 4 <br> Translator | | | |
| **Zhang We** 5 <br> Director of Resources | | | |

Score **2 points** for each name you remember   **Your score** _____

---

Your score    /75     **60–75 GOLD**

**30–59 SILVER**

**0–29 BRONZE**

You are brilliant at remembering names and faces, and are probably blessed with a good memory overall. Hone your skills by practising techniques like the three-step booster.

You could improve your memory for names and faces. Check out the Challenge on page 178 and keep working on your name–face associations.

You could be inconveniencing and embarrassing yourself with your poor memory for names and faces. Try the Challenge on page 178 and then go back and work through the exercises, with special attention to the techniques.

 Turn to page 178 for the Challenge.

## CHAPTER 3

# EVERYDAY ELEPHANT

## EVERYDAY CHALLENGES

# Everyday elephant

In the modern world there is a host of commonplace tasks and data to remember – the sort of things our memories struggle to cope with. To master the mundane requires a special blend of short- and long-term memory boosters.

## QUESTIONNAIRE
Complete this quick questionnaire to evaluate your baseline performance in this area.

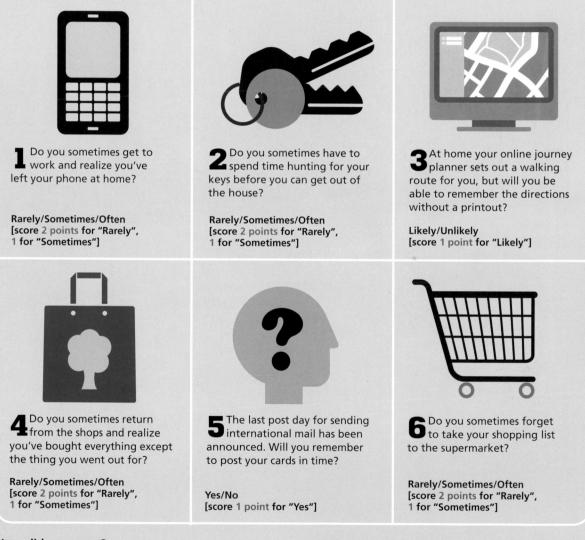

**1** Do you sometimes get to work and realize you've left your phone at home?

Rarely/Sometimes/Often
[score 2 points for "Rarely", 1 for "Sometimes"]

**2** Do you sometimes have to spend time hunting for your keys before you can get out of the house?

Rarely/Sometimes/Often
[score 2 points for "Rarely", 1 for "Sometimes"]

**3** At home your online journey planner sets out a walking route for you, but will you be able to remember the directions without a printout?

Likely/Unlikely
[score 1 point for "Likely"]

**4** Do you sometimes return from the shops and realize you've bought everything except the thing you went out for?

Rarely/Sometimes/Often
[score 2 points for "Rarely", 1 for "Sometimes"]

**5** The last post day for sending international mail has been announced. Will you remember to post your cards in time?

Yes/No
[score 1 point for "Yes"]

**6** Do you sometimes forget to take your shopping list to the supermarket?

Rarely/Sometimes/Often
[score 2 points for "Rarely", 1 for "Sometimes"]

**How did you score?**

**0–3:** Your memory for everyday tasks is weak. Fortunately this chapter is here to help – practise the techniques and work on the exercises.

**4–7:** Your memory for everyday tasks is average. Sharpen it by working on the exercises in this chapter.
**8–10:** You have a good memory for everyday tasks. This chapter will help you maintain this level of performance.

## 1 SHOPPING TEST

How much of your shopping can you remember without taking a list? Study the items on the right for 30 seconds. Now cover them up, list eight flowers, and then write down as many of the items as you can recall.

1  _M_

2  _E_

3  _W_

4  _Sh._

5  _C_

6  _P_

7  _St_

8  _B_

8/8: 1 point  Your score _____

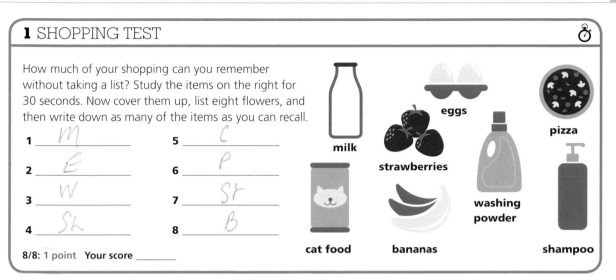

milk

eggs

pizza

strawberries

cat food

bananas

washing powder

shampoo

## TECHNIQUE: MEMORY HOUSE SYSTEM

The memory house is a mnemonic device (an aide mémoire) where you picture the layout of a house, place items on your list in the rooms, and create a memorable visual linking the item with the room. For example, below is a house and in each room is a memorable association to an item on a shopping list: spaghetti, lamb chops, toilet roll, soap, tuna, and wine. Study the house for 2 minutes, then cover it, wait 5 minutes, and write the list on a separate piece of paper.

Attic: girl with spaghetti hair

Bedroom: lamb in bed

Bathroom: soap in the bath

Living room: toilet roll on sofa

Kitchen: tuna fishing

Cellar: gorilla collecting wine

## 2 DIY MEMORY HOUSE

Practise the memory house system using the house below. Imagine the items from the list in the rooms in striking scenarios. Once you've finished, cover the house and list, and wait 2 minutes before trying to recall the list.

oranges
washing-up liquid
baked beans
cake
candles
tea bags
frozen peas

1  _____

2  _____

3  _____

4  _____

5  _____

6  _____

7  _____

7/7: 1 point
Your score _____

**TECHNIQUE: LINK SYSTEM**

The link system is another technique that uses strong imagery to make memorable associations. Items you want to remember are linked together in unusual and striking ways. Below is an example of how you might visualize, link, and remember three items on your shopping list.

**fish** **bacon** **bagels**

On your shopping list you need to remember these three items: fish, bacon, bagels.

**Step 1**
Create a memorable image for each item: a fish with hands, bacon dancing, bagels as balloons.

**Step 2**
Now link the three images into one single memorable visualization: the fish holding the bagel balloons and dancing with the bacon.

## 3 LINK LOVIN'

Let's work on the link system some more. On your shopping list are lemons, chocolate, milk, bread, and carrots. Below is a memorable image for each of these – can you think of one memorable scenario linking all five items? Now cover the images, list eight African countries, then try to remember your scenario and use it to recall the items on your list. Write them down on the note paper provided.

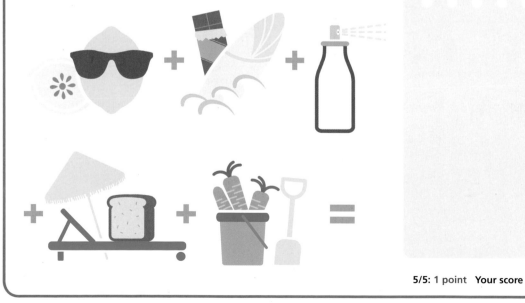

**5/5: 1 point Your score** _____

## 4 LINK LIFE

You can also use the link system to remember lists of household chores or appointments. Write or sketch link visualizations for each set of images below, then cover them and come back 5 minutes later to test your recall for the link.

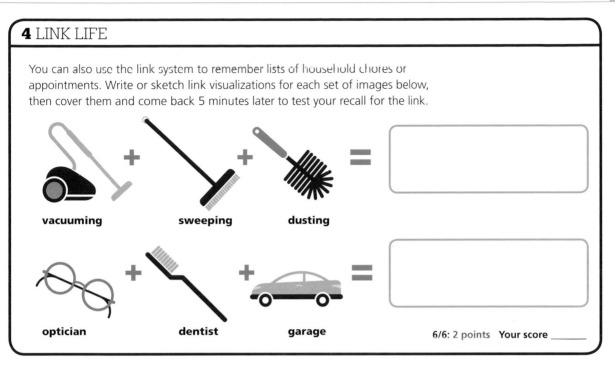

**vacuuming**  +  **sweeping**  +  **dusting**  =

**optician**  +  **dentist**  +  **garage**  =

6/6: 2 points   Your score _____

---

**TECHNIQUE: ACRONYMS ASSEMBLE**

An acronym is a word formed from the initial letters of a series of words. For example, WHO is an acronym for World Health Organization. You can use the initials of items on a list you need to remember to make a memorable acronym. Suppose an acronym of your shopping list spelled out TYGRR: you could then also use a tiger as the basis for a visualization. Try turning the initials of these items you need for a picnic into a memorable acronym.

**plates, apples, basket, utensils, bread, cupcakes, wine, ice pack**

## 5 ACRONYM ANTICS

Practise the acronym technique by using it to generate a memorable acronym for this list of things you need to get from the DIY store. Pick one that suggests a striking image, fix it in your mind, then cover the list. Write down eight vegetables and then try to recall the list.

**hammer, underlay, nails, glue, oil, file, tape measure, paint**

_____

_____

_____

_____

_____

_____

_____

**8/8: 2 points 7/8: 1 point**

**Your score** _____

_____

## TECHNIQUE: ACROSTIC TACTICS

An acrostic is a phrase, verse, or sentence where the initial letters of each word on a list or in a sequence spell out a word to combine together into a sentence you can easily remember. You can then use this sentence (or acrostic) to remind you of the words you are trying to remember. For instance, Hurry Up The Beach is Lovely could stand for a list of things to take to the beach: hat, umbrella, towel, books, and lotion. Try making an acrostic to remind you of the ingredients you need for a cake:

**flour, sugar, milk, butter, eggs, lemons, nutmeg**

## 6 ACROSTIC SLEEPOVER

Your child is having a sleepover: make sure you don't forget anything by coming up with an acrostic for the items on the right. Then cover the items and your acrostic, name eight marine creatures, and then using your acrostic see if you can recall the items you need to remember for the sleepover.

1 _____

2 _____

3 _____

4 _____

5 _____

6 _____

7 _____

**7/7: 2 points  6/7: 1 point**

**Your score** _____

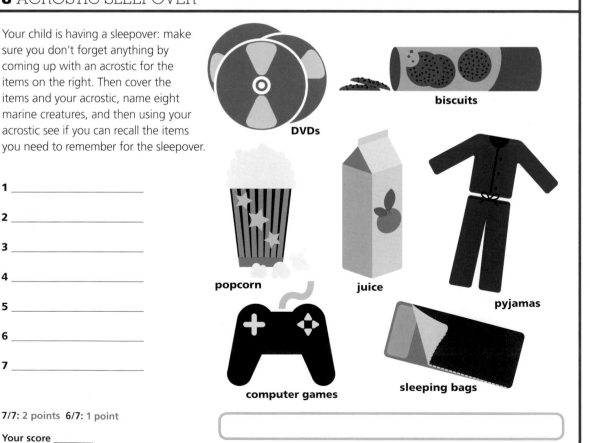

DVDs

biscuits

popcorn

juice

pyjamas

computer games

sleeping bags

## 7 ACROSTIC CHRISTMAS LIST

A relative has given you her Christmas wish list. Make sure you don't forget any of the gifts on the list by coming up with a memorable acrostic from an arrangement of the first letters of the items below. Cover the list and your acrostic, wait 5 minutes, and then try to recall the list.

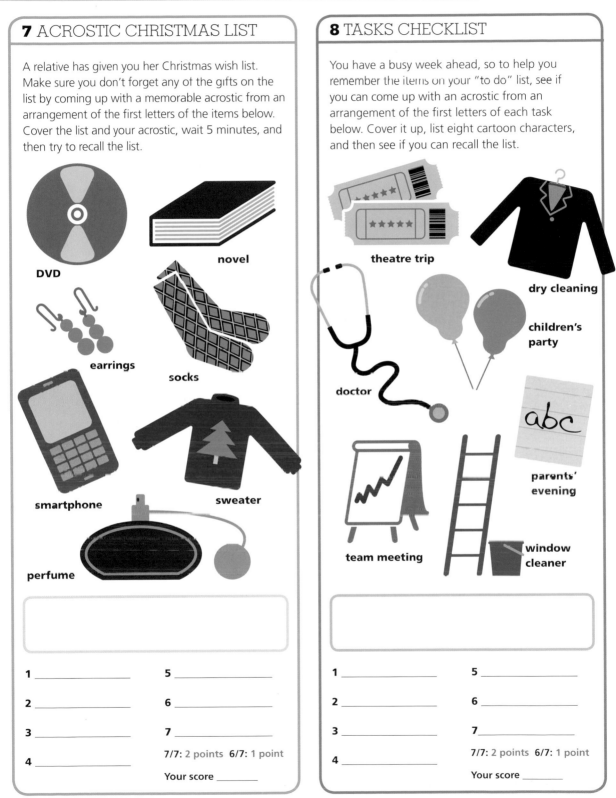

**DVD**

**novel**

**earrings**

**socks**

**smartphone**

**sweater**

**perfume**

1 _____  5 _____

2 _____  6 _____

3 _____  7 _____

4 _____

**7/7: 2 points  6/7: 1 point**

**Your score** _____

## 8 TASKS CHECKLIST

You have a busy week ahead, so to help you remember the items on your "to do" list, see if you can come up with an acrostic from an arrangement of the first letters of each task below. Cover it up, list eight cartoon characters, and then see if you can recall the list.

**theatre trip**

**dry cleaning**

**children's party**

**doctor**

**abc**

**parents' evening**

**team meeting**

**window cleaner**

1 _____  5 _____

2 _____  6 _____

3 _____  7 _____

4 _____

**7/7: 2 points  6/7: 1 point**

**Your score** _____

49

A peg system is a mnemonic where you create a series of striking images that you know off by heart (your "pegs"). You can create a visualization linking your pegs to the things that you need to remember (such as the items on a shopping list or a list of household chores). The theory is that because you already know your pegs, it is easy to recall the visualizations linked to them and therefore you can remember the items on the list. Once you have formed and memorized your peg images, you have a ready-made and widely applicable toolkit for use in forming memorable imagery-based associations with items on any list you need to remember. There are many possible peg systems. Here, the alphabet peg system is shown and pegs have been created for the first three letters of the alphabet. Follow the steps and see if you can come up with your own memorable pegs for the whole alphabet.

**Items to remember:**
oranges
pasta
cheese

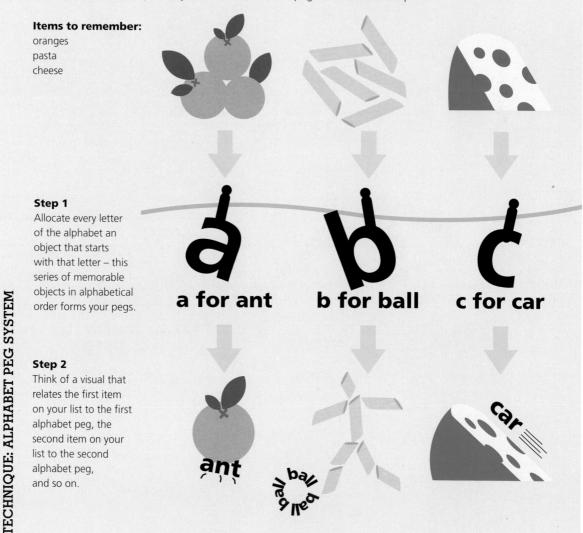

**TECHNIQUE: ALPHABET PEG SYSTEM**

**Step 1**
Allocate every letter of the alphabet an object that starts with that letter – this series of memorable objects in alphabetical order forms your pegs.

**a for ant**  **b for ball**  **c for car**

**Step 2**
Think of a visual that relates the first item on your list to the first alphabet peg, the second item on your list to the second alphabet peg, and so on.

**Step 3**
When you need to remember a list, work through your alphabet pegs and each respective visualization to help you recall the items on it. The key is to learn your alphabet pegs; then visualizations should be easily recalled.

## 9 ALPHABET PEG PRACTICE

Use your own alphabet pegs to memorize the items you need to pack for a holiday. For instance, if your peg for "d" is "dog" you could imagine the corresponding item on the list – your passport – open to the photo page with a passport photo of a dog. Try applying the alphabet peg system to the whole of the list on the right, then cover it, wait 5 minutes, and see if you can recall all the items in order.

**money**
**tickets**
**guidebook**
**passport**
**sunglasses**
**sun cream**
**flip flops**
**toothbrush**
**camera**
**phrase book**

1 _____
2 _____
3 _____
4 _____
5 _____
6 _____
7 _____
8 _____
9 _____
10 _____

**10/10: 2 points  8–9: 1 point  Your score** _____

## 10 MORE ALPHABET PEG PRACTICE

Practise your alphabet peg technique again by using it to memorize a list of sights you want to see when you visit Sydney. For instance, if your peg for "c" is "car", create a visual in your head for the corresponding item on your list – perhaps the fish in the aquarium (representing Sydney Aquarium) driving a car. Try this for the whole list below, cover it, name five Australian cities, then try to recall all the sights in order.

**Sydney Opera House**
**Royal Botanic Gardens**
**Sydney Aquarium**
**Museum of Contemporary Art**
**Sydney Harbour Bridge**

**The Rocks**
**Taronga Zoo**
**Circular Quay**
**Batemans Bay**
**Jenolan Caves**

1 _____
2 _____
3 _____
4 _____
5 _____
6 _____
7 _____
8 _____
9 _____
10 _____

**10/10: 2 points  8–9: 1 point  Your score** _____

Another peg system you can apply to help everyday memory of lists and tasks is the rhyming number peg system. Here, your pegs are numbers instead of letters. Attached to each number peg is a word that rhymes with that number. You can then associate the things on your list to your rhyming pegs.

**Items to remember:**
oranges
pasta
cheese

**Step 1**
Think of a word that rhymes with the number of the peg. For example, 1 could be sun, 2 could be shoe, 3 could be sea, and so on.

**Step 2**
Relate each item on your list to the corresponding peg number. So, if the first thing on your list is oranges, apply oranges to the number 1 peg by linking the item to the rhyming word to create a memorable image. For example, you could visualize an orange as the sun. Do the same with the rest of the items on the list.

**Step 3**
When you need to remember your list, work through your rhyming number pegs and their associated visuals to help you recall the items on it.

## 11 RHYMING NUMBER PEG PRACTICE

Practise your rhyming number peg system by applying it to a list of household chores. Assign the chores to your number rhymes in sequence, making striking associations. For instance, if your rhyme for "8" is "plate", you could visualize a clean bath full of plates. When you've visualized the whole list, cover it and wait 5 minutes. Now try to recall the list of chores in order.

**mop kitchen floor**
**take out rubbish**
**clean fridge**
**empty recycling**
**fill up salt cellar**
**mow lawn**
**change sheets**
**clean bath**

1 _____

2 _____

3 _____

4 _____

5 _____

6 _____

7 _____

8 _____

**8/8: 2 points  7/8: 1 point**

**Your score _____**

## 12 CHUNK THAT LIST

As we saw in Chapter 1, chunking – splitting items into related groups – is a handy shortcut for remembering things. Previously, you sorted the items into pairs. Now, group items into categories of more than two. Divide these school items into three groups based on where the items will go – sports bag, lunch box, and school bag. Cover it up, name eight insects, and then try to recall the list, writing each item in the relevant place.

**trainers**
**socks**
**racket**
**sweatband**
**apple**
**fruit juice**
**sandwich**
**grapes**
**homework**
**textbooks**
**pencil case**
**calculator**

**12/12:** 2 points  **10–11:** 1 point

**Your score** _____

## 13 SUPERMARKET SWEEP

Another way of chunking is to divide a shopping list according to the aisles of the supermarket you will need to visit. Assign each of these items to the relevant aisle at the supermarket – fruit and vegetables, freezer, or drinks – then cover the list and name eight breeds of dogs. Then try to remember the list by recalling which aisle you will find each item on.

**lemonade**
**oven chips**
**grapes**
**bottled water**
**potatoes**
**ice cream**
**leeks**
**blackcurrant cordial**
**ice cubes**
**lager**
**water melon**
**frozen prawns**

**12/12 items:** 2 points  **10–11:** 1 point   **Your score** _____

# 14 MOON STREET

Remembering directions can be difficult and it can help to use the names of streets to suggest memorable images. Try memorizing this list of directions, then cover and retest yourself after waiting 5 minutes.

Left at **Nightingale Avenue**

Straight on at **Moon Street**

Right at **Floral Lane**

Right again at **Farm Fields**

Straight on down **Frenchman's Row**

Left at **The Cut**

Right at **Wall Street**

1 _____     5 _____

2 _____     6 _____

3 _____     7 _____

4 _____     **7/7: 1 point**

                      **Your score _____**

# 15 COMPASS ROSE

Add to your direction visualization a system for remembering left–right orientation. For instance, a system based on a compass that equates West with an appropriate image (such as a cowboy) and uses that as a mnemonic image for left. East becomes right, North means go straight on and South means double back. Can you come up with images for these?

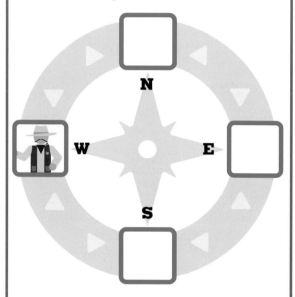

Now try combining this system with images suggested by place names in this sequence of directions. Once you have an image for each direction, cover the list and write your name backwards. Now see if you can recall all five directions using the images you created.

**1** Turn left onto Tower Street
**2** Go straight across at the junction with Hangman's Hill
**3** Turn right onto Cloudman's Road
**4** Turn left onto Weasley Gardens
**5** Go straight across at St Paul's Square

1 _____     4 _____

2 _____     5 _____

3 _____     **5/5: 1 point**

                      **Your score _____**

## 16 LEFT AND RIGHT

A flurry of directions can be hard to remember. Turn the lefts and rights into an acrostic by combining pairs of directions into the basis for words. For instance, left followed by right (LR) becomes **LiRa**. Right followed by right (RR) becomes **RoaRing**. Try turning directions into words with the series of directions below, then cover the directions, list eight clothing items, and trace out a path on the grid beginning at "start".

**Right, left; Left, right; Right, left; Right, right**

Where did you end up? _____

Answer on page 180

Right place: score 1 point   Your score _____

stables

guitar shop

temple          church

park

stamp museum

city farm

fountain          flower garden

butterfly centre

tall house

↑ START

## 17 WAYPOINTS

Chunking is a great technique for making a long set of directions easier to remember. Essentially this means breaking down your journey into sections, like following a series of waypoints. So rather than remembering how to get all the way from Berry Road to Garfield Place, you remember how to get from Berry Road to C Street, then C Street to Jefferson Square, and so on. Chunk this list, then cover it and try to navigate the map.

**1** East on Berry Road
**2** Fourth right onto Brick Lane
**3** First right onto C Street
**4** Cross over the crossroads
**5** Turn left onto Diwan Avenue
**6** Second right into Jefferson Square
**7** Across the square and up Sharma Heights
**8** Third right onto Garfield Place

How many directions did you remember? 8/8: **2 points** 7/8: **1 point**   Your score _____

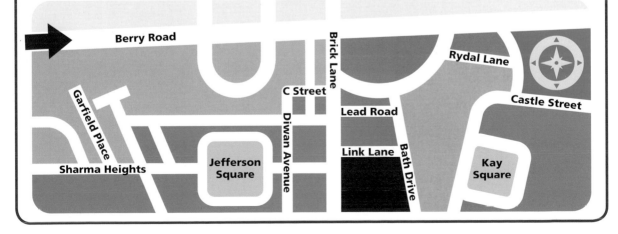

## 18 KEY FINDER

Remembering, let alone finding, keys is an everyday challenge for many people. Test your key memory with this quick quiz: where are these keys right now?

1 _____

2 _____

3 _____

4 _____

**1. Front door key**    **2. Car key**    **3. Garden door key**    **4. Bike lock key**

## 19 KEYS TO THE KINGDOM

Improve your memory for key location by building striking associations between each key and where you keep it. Below are four images to help you remember four different locations. Visualize them for 30 seconds, cover them, name eight rivers, then try to remember where all four keys are.

1 _____

2 _____

3 _____

4 _____

**1. In flower vase**    **2. On hook next to umbrella stand**    **3. On top of wardrobe with old boxes**    **4. In drawer with sewing kit**

**1 point** for remembering all locations   Your score _____

## 20 KEY CREATIVITY

Try coming up with your own visual locations for keys. Here are four locations – for each one write or sketch a memorable visual link. Then cover and come back after counting up your score so far for this chapter. Can you remember all four locations?

1 _____

2 _____

3 _____

4 _____

**2. In jar on kitchen counter**

**1. On top of frame of door leading onto garden**

**3. In drawer in hall bureau with passports and foreign money**

**4. On hook by front door next to boots and shoes**

**4/4: 1 point** Your score _____

**TIP**

Make a home for your keys. If you always put your keys in the same place you will never have to look for them! Pick a good spot – for example, a hook in the hallway – and make a point of always hanging your keys there when you come in. If you forget, go and do it as soon as you remember. Soon it will become a habit and your keys will never be lost again.

Your score          /40          **30–40 GOLD**          **10–29 SILVER**          **0–9 BRONZE**

| | | |
|---|---|---|
| Impressive – your memory is in good shape for everyday tasks. Keep practising visualization and association skills to keep up the high level of performance. | Your memory is average when it comes to everyday tasks. Check out the Challenge on page 178, and go back and work on some of the tips. | Poor memory hampers your performance on everyday tasks. Try out the Challenge and then go back and work through the puzzles again. |

★ Turn to page 178 for the Challenge

CHAPTER 4
# WHERE'S MY CAR?
## MEDIUM-TERM MEMORY

# Where's my car?

Somewhere between short- and long-term memory is a stage where information is being laid down, but is not yet fully encoded. This is medium-term memory (MTM). Anything you have remembered for more than a minute but less than a week fits into this category.

## QUESTIONNAIRE
Use this quick quiz to get an instant rating of your MTM skills.

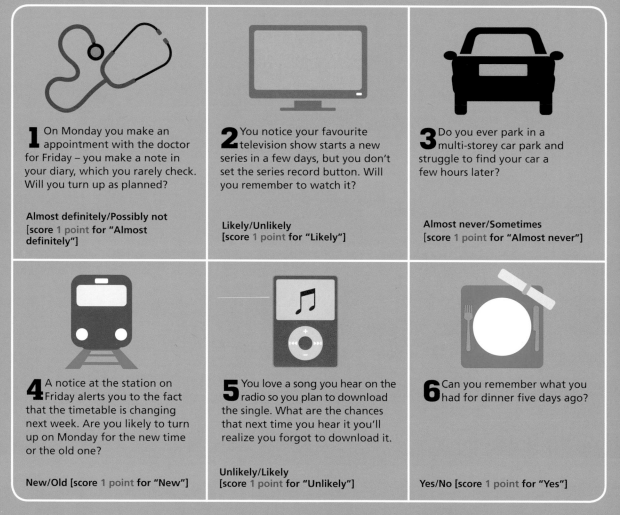

**1** On Monday you make an appointment with the doctor for Friday – you make a note in your diary, which you rarely check. Will you turn up as planned?

**Almost definitely/Possibly not [score 1 point for "Almost definitely"]**

**2** You notice your favourite television show starts a new series in a few days, but you don't set the series record button. Will you remember to watch it?

**Likely/Unlikely [score 1 point for "Likely"]**

**3** Do you ever park in a multi-storey car park and struggle to find your car a few hours later?

**Almost never/Sometimes [score 1 point for "Almost never"]**

**4** A notice at the station on Friday alerts you to the fact that the timetable is changing next week. Are you likely to turn up on Monday for the new time or the old one?

**New/Old [score 1 point for "New"]**

**5** You love a song you hear on the radio so you plan to download the single. What are the chances that next time you hear it you'll realize you forgot to download it.

**Unlikely/Likely [score 1 point for "Unlikely"]**

**6** Can you remember what you had for dinner five days ago?

**Yes/No [score 1 point for "Yes"]**

### How did you score?
**0–2:** A poor MTM means you are likely to be forgetting things from one day to the next, which is especially trying. There are lots of tips in this chapter to help you.
**3–4:** Your MTM is average, which means you would benefit from improvements. Work through the exercises in this chapter, paying close attention to the techniques, and see how you get on.
**5–6:** Your MTM is strong, and you are unlikely to miss appointments, forget arrangements, or lose cars. Hone your abilities with these exercises, and practise new strategies to maintain your MTM performance.

# 1 CALL HISTORY

A good way to stretch your MIM is to see if you can recall (without electronic aids) the people who called you most recently on your mobile phone. List the names of your last five callers below.

1 _____

2 _____

3 _____

4 _____

5 _____

**Score 1 point for each caller remembered**

**Your score** _____

# 2 DINNER DIARY

A good test of MIM is whether you can recall what you ate for dinner recently. Can you fill in this dinner diary?

What did you have for dinner...

**yesterday** _____ Score 1 point

**2 days ago** _____ Score 1 point

**3 days ago** _____ Score 1 point

**4 days ago** _____ Score 1 point

**5 days ago** _____ Score 2 points

**Your score** _____

# 3 AD BUSTER

Stretch your MTM some more by seeing if you can remember adverts you have seen on television. When watching TV, write down the first five adverts you see, then see if you can recall them at the same time the next day.

1 _____

2 _____

3 _____

4 _____

5 _____

**Score 1 point for each advert you remembered**

**Your score** _____

The journey method is a peg system to help you remember things on a list. The stages of a journey (either real-life or fictional) are the pegs. Once you have decided on your journey and its various stages, you can then link each stage to an item on your list by creating a visualization linking the two. Below, for example, the first stage of a journey is passing the gates of horn, which are guarded by griffons – this is your peg to which you link the first item you need to remember on your list. Practice is key with the journey method, so to begin, try to remember these six fantasy journey stages as your pegs, and recall them after 5 minutes.

**1** The gates of horn, guarded by griffons

**2** The forest of fear, infested by goblins

**3** The meadow of sleep, full of poppies

**4** The bottomless chasm, crossed by a rope bridge

**5** The fortress of bronze, with a custard moat

**6** The waterfall of ice, filled with red fish

**TECHNIQUE: JOURNEY METHOD**

## 4 JOURNEY METHOD PRACTICE

Use your journey pegs (either your own or the example journey, left) to remember the six tasks listed below. For each one, a striking visual link between the item and the journey stage has been made. For example, for "pick up granny", the first item, you could imagine granny being carried away by a griffon. When you've understood and memorized the visualizations, cover the list, name 8 types of fruit, then see how many of the tasks on the list you can remember.

**1** Pick up granny

**2** Call dentist

**3** Get present

**4** Get tyres checked

**5** Call Barbara

**6** Water houseplants

1 _____  4 _____

2 _____  5 _____

3 _____  6 _____

**6/6: 1 point**

**Your score** _____

## 5 CAR PARK PANIC

Use the journey method to memorize where you have parked your car. Once you've made your visualizations, cover the list, and come back in 5 minutes and locate the correct bay.

You parked in: **Green level, Area E, Bay 13**

**Correct bay remembered: 1 point   Your score** _____

## 6 THERE AND BACK AGAIN

You've just started a new job and you need to learn the new commute. Use the journey method to help you remember the landmarks along the route. Cover the list of landmarks, name eight birds, then try to recall your new route.

**1** Train station
**2** Town hall
**3** Police station
**4** Swimming pool
**5** Park
**6** Roundabout

1 _____

2 _____

3 _____

4 _____

5 _____

6 _____

**6/6: 1 point   Your score** _____

## 7 FLOOR PLAN

You could also use the rooms of a multi-storey building, such as a college, for your journey pegs. Imagine you are a student and have to remember the list of textbooks you need to buy for your course. Create a memorable visualization between the room and the book title. Cover the list of textbooks, name eight Disney films, then see if you can recall the titles.

1 _____       4 _____

2 _____       5 _____

3 _____       6 _____

**6/6: 1 point**

**Your score** _____

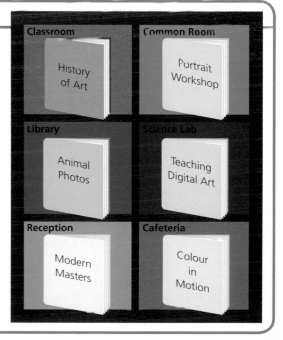

## TECHNIQUE: DAYS OF THE WEEK PEG SYSTEM

The days of the week make another good basis for a peg system. The pegs are the individual days (Monday, Tuesday, and so on), and each peg is linked to a memorable visual. The visual could, for example, be something that stems from the word itself, such as the spelling, look, or pronunciation of the word. You could link Monday to the moon; Tuesday to twins ("two" sounds similar to "Tue"); Wednesday to a wedding cake (the "wed" of Wednesday); Thursday to a hammer (the shape of a capital "T"); Friday to a frying pan (the pronunciation of "Fri"); Saturday to a chair (you have "sat" in a chair); and Sunday to the sun. Once you have learnt your visuals for each peg, you can then use them to help you remember events taking place on a particular day in the week ahead. Think of a visualization linking the event you need to remember to the day on which it occurs. For example, if you have a geography examination on Tuesday, you could think of an image with twins holding the Earth. Memorize your own pegs, or the ones given here, before trying the following puzzles.

**MONDAY** — Violin lesson
**TUESDAY** — Geography exam
**WEDNESDAY** — Tennis match
**THURSDAY** — Visit library
**FRIDAY** — Cinema club

## 8 CLASS TIME

Imagine you've just started a new year at school – classes start every morning at 9am, but can you remember which class to turn up for first on which day? Use the weekday peg system above to create visualizations for which lesson takes place on which day. List eight mountains, then test yourself.

**Mon:** History
**Tue:** Spanish
**Wed:** Chemistry
**Thu:** Biology
**Fri:** Economics

### Timetable

| | |
|---|---|
| **Mon** | _____ |
| **Tue** | _____ |
| **Wed** | _____ |
| **Thu** | _____ |
| **Fri** | _____ |

4/4: 1 point    Your score _____

## TIP

An exercise to stretch your MTM into long-term memory is to take a trip in your mind's eye down a street or route that you know well – your route home from work, for example. Try to remember and visualize all the major landmarks on the way, and estimate the time it takes to walk between them. Name the streets, shops, and natural features you go past. Try to make your visualization as detailed as possible, with colours, textures, sounds, and smells.

# 9 DAYS OF THE WEEK PEG PRACTICE

It is Sunday evening and you need to remember various activities taking place on specific days in the coming week. Use your days of the week pegs to create visualizations to help you remember what is taking place on which day. On Monday morning, see if you can remember your itinerary for the week.

**Mon:** Meeting with architects
**Tue:** Choosing carpets
**Wed:** Football match

**Thu:** Pick up boss from airport
**Fri:** Deadline for report

**Sat:** Going to the theatre
**Sun:** Family lunch

Mon _____

Tue _____

Wed _____

Thu _____

Fri _____

Sat _____

Sun _____

**7/7: 2 points 6/7: 1 point   Your score ____**

# 10 INTERVIEW WEEK

You can use memorable aspects of an appointment itself to make striking associations with your weekday pegs. You have five different interviews set up. Work through the names on the right and assign associations between the names and your pegs. Cover them up and after 5 minutes see if you can remember who you are seeing on which day and the company's name.

Mon _____

Tue _____

Wed _____

Thu _____

Fri _____

**5/5: 2 points  4/5: 1 point   Your score _____**

**Monday:** Brenda at **Black Lagoon Ltd**

**Wednesday:** Tariq at **Banner House**

**Tuesday:** Darren at **Tower Lights**

**Thursday:** Phillip at **Shell Place**

**Friday:** Ellie at **Berry & Sons**

For remembering specific times, or just as a generic peg system, a clock-face-based series of pegs is useful. Here the pegs are the hour numbers on a clock. Each peg is linked to a memorable visualization relating to that number or to the position on the clock face. For example, the hour 12 on the clock face ties in with North, or the hour 4 can be linked to a square, which has four sides. You then create a visualization between the hour peg of the appointment time you need to remember and the actual appointment. For example, if you needed to remember a doctor's appointment for 12 o'clock, you could visualize a needle pointing North. See if you can commit to memory these example hour visualizations, and also try to come up with your own version. Cover the clocks and name eight American states. Now test your memory of the pegs.

## 11 DIARY TREK

Can you use the clock peg system to memorize these seven appointments? Study them for 2 minutes, and when you're finished, cover them up, and think of five dinosaurs. Now fill in the blank diary spaces on the right.

**9am** _____

**10am** _____

**11am** _____

**12am** _____

**2pm** _____

**3pm** _____

**4pm** _____

**9am:** Marketing team meeting

**10am:** Sales pitch

**11am:** Quarterly results due

**12am:** TV interview

**2pm:** Partners' meeting

**3pm:** Interview receptionist candidates

**4pm:** Team drinks

**7/7: 2 points**
**6/7: 1 point**

**Your score** _____

## 12 NOW SHOWING

You're trying to plan a night at the cinema but you only get a quick glance at the showing times for your local cinemas. Can you memorize which film is on at what time and where, in under 2 minutes? Then cover the list, think of five comedy films, and test your recall.

**5pm:** The Red Rose at the Film House

**7pm:** Santa vs Aliens at the Roxy

**8pm:** Lords of the Air at the Empire

**11pm:** Too Many Cooks at the Curzon

**Score 1 point** for each showing time you correctly recalled   **Your score** _____

## 13 MEDICATION MNEMONIC

A course of medication can involve a complicated timetable for taking pills. Use a clock peg system to help. Study the schedule below for 1 minute, cover it, write down your five favourite films, then test yourself.

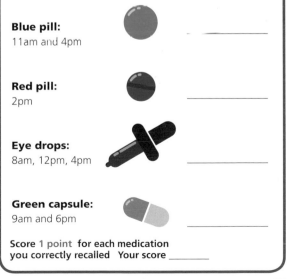

**Blue pill:**
11am and 4pm

_____

**Red pill:**
2pm

_____

**Eye drops:**
8am, 12pm, 4pm

_____

**Green capsule:**
9am and 6pm

_____

**Score 1 point** for each medication you correctly recalled   **Your score** _____

## 14 PROGRAMME REMINDER

Combining clock and weekday pegs can ensure you never miss your favourite TV show again. For example, if you want to remember to watch a period drama, and it is on at 7pm every Monday, you could visualize the sun setting (your hour peg for 7 o'clock) over the moon (your weekday peg for Monday). Look at the schedule of programmes below for 2 minutes and combine your visualizations for the weekday and hour, then cover them all. List five green vegetables, then test your recall of the programmes and the times they are showing.

**Mondays 8pm:**
Family Circle

**Tuesdays 7pm:**
Horse World

**Wednesdays 8am:**
Global News

1 _____

2 _____

3 _____

4 _____

5 _____

6 _____

**Thursdays 9pm:**
Birdwatch America

**Saturdays 10am:**
The Chef Show

**Sundays 2pm:**
Eden Gardens

**6/6:** 2 points
**5/6:** 1 point

**Your score** _____

## 15 FESTIVAL FUN TIMES

You're at a music festival and you don't want to miss any of your favourite bands. Using the combined clock and weekday peg system, memorize the line-up, then list five radio stations, before writing down which band is on when.

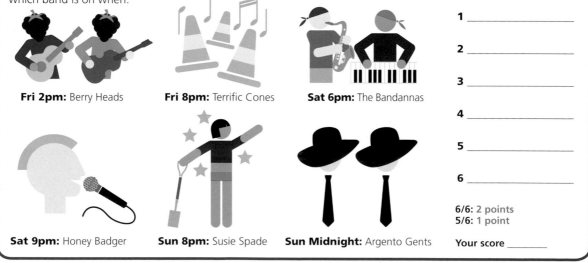

**Fri 2pm:** Berry Heads

**Fri 8pm:** Terrific Cones

**Sat 6pm:** The Bandannas

1 _____

2 _____

3 _____

4 _____

5 _____

6 _____

**Sat 9pm:** Honey Badger

**Sun 8pm:** Susie Spade

**Sun Midnight:** Argento Gents

**6/6:** 2 points
**5/6:** 1 point

**Your score** _____

## 16 OLYMPIC ROUND-UP

There's a big week of Olympic sporting action ahead and you don't miss your favourite events. Using your combined clock and weekday peg system, can you memorize which sports are on when? Study the sports and times below for 1 minute, then cover them and name five sports played with a ball, before testing your recall.

**Friday 9am:**
Men's 200m hurdles

**Wednesday 10.30am:**
Men's tennis

**Thursday 1pm:**
Women's 100m swimming

**Thursday 6pm:**
Women's shotput

**Monday 11am:**
Women's archery

**Sunday 7pm:**
Men's heavyweight judo

1 _____
2 _____
3 _____
4 _____
5 _____
6 _____

**6/6:** 1 point

**Your score** _____

## 17 CRUISE CONTROL

There are lots of onboard events and activities on offer during your week-long cruise holiday, and you don't want to miss any of them. Can you memorize the timetable below using the combined clock and weekday peg system? Give yourself 2 minutes of memorizing, then name five seas, and test for recall.

**Sunday 8am:** Captain's welcome talk and ship orientation

**Monday 12 noon:** pool aerobics

**Tuesday 11pm:** cabaret and revue in the theatre

**Wednesday 2pm:** giant quoits game on deck

**Thursday 6am:** early bird snorkelling on the reef

**Friday 10pm:** karaoke in the Captain's Lounge

**Saturday 5pm:** advanced knots with the Quartermaster

1 _____
2 _____
3 _____
4 _____
5 _____
6 _____
7 _____

**7/7:** 4 points  **6/7:** 3 points
**5/7:** 2 points  **4/7:** 1 point

**Your score** _____

---

Your score        /50

 **40–50 GOLD**

Your MTM is well prepared for the challenges of everyday life, and if you can make a habit of practising some of the tips and strategies covered in this chapter, your MTM will stay in tip-top condition.

 **20–39 SILVER**

You've given your MTM a good workout but you could benefit from improvements in all areas. Read the Challenge on page 178, and go back and try again exercises where you struggled.

**0–19 BRONZE**

Your MTM is causing you problems. Try the Challenge on page 178, and go back and work through the exercises again.

 Turn to page 178 for the Challenge.

## CHAPTER 5

# I KNOW WHAT I DID LAST SUMMER

## LONG-TERM MEMORY

# I know what I did last summer

Long-term memory (LTM) comes in many forms: memory of events that have happened in your life is known as biographical memory; recall of isolated facts requires semantic memory; and knowledge of skills, such as tying your shoelaces, is known as procedural memory.

## QUESTIONNAIRE
Use this quick quiz to get an instant readout of your LTM status.

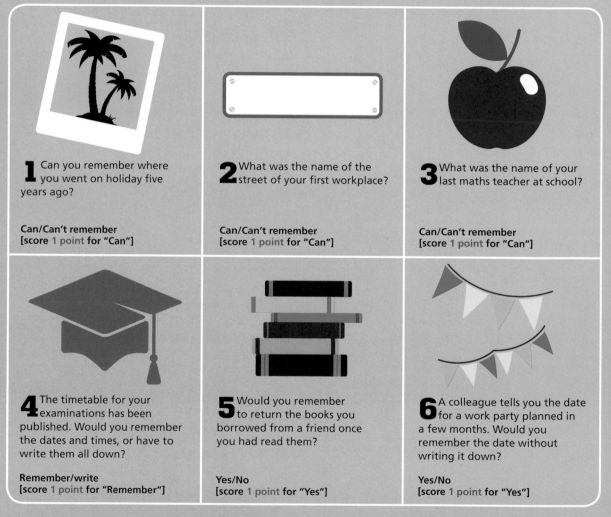

**1** Can you remember where you went on holiday five years ago?

**Can/Can't remember**
[score 1 point for "Can"]

**2** What was the name of the street of your first workplace?

**Can/Can't remember**
[score 1 point for "Can"]

**3** What was the name of your last maths teacher at school?

**Can/Can't remember**
[score 1 point for "Can"]

**4** The timetable for your examinations has been published. Would you remember the dates and times, or have to write them all down?

**Remember/write**
[score 1 point for "Remember"]

**5** Would you remember to return the books you borrowed from a friend once you had read them?

**Yes/No**
[score 1 point for "Yes"]

**6** A colleague tells you the date for a work party planned in a few months. Would you remember the date without writing it down?

**Yes/No**
[score 1 point for "Yes"]

### How did you score?
**0–2:** Your biographical memory is weak. The exercises in this chapter will help you to expand your memory, and the techniques will help you improve it in the future.
**3–4:** You have an average biographical memory, which nevertheless means you could be forgetting important episodes. Work through the chapter to get a clearer picture of the strengths and gaps.
**5–6:** Your biographical memory is excellent; you should enjoy completing the exercises in this chapter, and along the way you may pick up tips to help keep this faculty in top condition.

## 1 WONDER YEARS

Despite what some people claim, everyone suffers from childhood amnesia: the loss of memories from the earliest years, before around age three to four. Let's probe the limits of your memory. In the spaces below, write down your five earliest memories.

## 2 TIMELINE

Let's go for a trip down memory lane with this timeline of life events. For each one rate your recall on a scale of 0 (it's a blank!) to 5 (total recall). Work out your overall score based on the categories you answered.

**Recall**

| | |
|---|---|
| _____ | First day at primary school |
| _____ | Reception classroom |
| _____ | Starting at secondary school |
| _____ | First date |
| _____ | Exam results in last year of sixth form |
| _____ | Passing your driving test |
| _____ | Graduation |
| _____ | First job |
| _____ | Wedding |
| _____ | Moving into first family home |
| _____ | Birth of first child |
| _____ | Retirement |

Total recall score _____

**To work out your overall grading, multiply your total recall score by 10. Then add up the number of categories you answered and multiply this by 5. Now divide the first answer by the second to work out the number of points you scored out of 10.**

Your score _____

## 3 FAMILY TREE

Your family history is an important part of your biographical makeup. Using the family tree below as an example, push your biographical memory to the limit by creating your own family tree on a separate piece of paper and seeing how far back you can go.

TECHNIQUE: EXPLORE THE SENSES

Even people for whom the biographical past is difficult to remember can find that once they start exploring their memories, things come flooding back. A useful strategy is to explore a memory one sense at a time. What could you smell? Were there any background noises? And so on. Below are some illustrated examples. Can you come up with your own sensory memories for these two travel experiences?

**First seaside holiday**

**First foreign trip**

## 4 POSTCARDS FROM THE PAST

Can you fill in your sensory memories for these events?

| last holiday | last road trip | 18th birthday | last restaurant visit |

For each event, score **2 points** if you filled in 5/5 categories, **1 point** if you filled in 4/5    Your score _____

It can be difficult to remember the names of old acquaintances and distant relatives. Use this technique to help boost your memory when you meet up with people again in years to come. Use a familiar cast of characters from a well-known story and create memorable visualizations linking the faces and names to the characters. Try out this example using Snow White and the Seven Dwarves to memorize the names of five friends. Create a memorable image for each, linking the individual to one of the characters, then cover the faces and after 5 minutes, recall your visualizations and see if you can remember the five names.

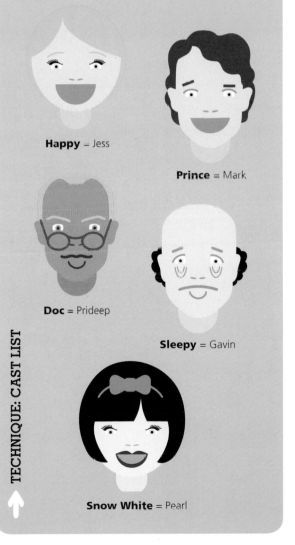

**Happy** – Jess

**Prince** = Mark

**Doc** = Prideep

**Sleepy** = Gavin

**Snow White** = Pearl

**TECHNIQUE: CAST LIST**

## 5 CASTING CALL

Can you come up with your own cast of characters to use as a visualization? For instance, you could use characters from famous films or books or comics. Using a line up of your own invention, take 3 minutes to link the names and features of the people below to characters in your cast. List five farm animals, then test your recall of their names.

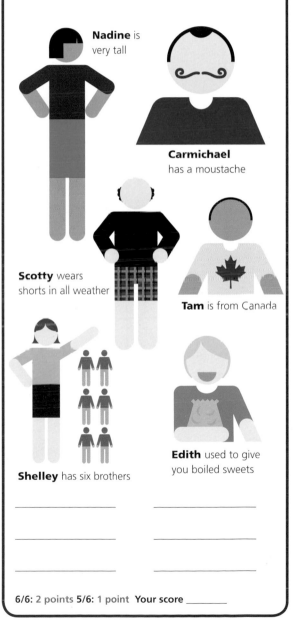

**Nadine** is very tall

**Carmichael** has a moustache

**Scotty** wears shorts in all weather

**Tam** is from Canada

**Shelley** has six brothers

**Edith** used to give you boiled sweets

_____    _____

_____    _____

_____    _____

6/6: 2 points 5/6: 1 point  **Your score** _____

When you commit dates and appointments to memory, it is similar to committing any other isolated fact to memory, and this uses your semantic memory. As with other peg systems, these calendar pegs help boost encoding and recall of semantic memory through use of vivid, memorable, and accessible images.

The months of the year make good pegs because they are a familiar sequence and help with recall of dates and appointments. Here are some suggested peg images for the months of the year relating to the season/name of the month itself. For example, if you want to remember that your office outing is in May, you can visualize the members of your team having a picnic in a field full of flowers. Memorize the list of 12 pegs below, cover them and write out the alphabet backwards, then see if you can recall them.

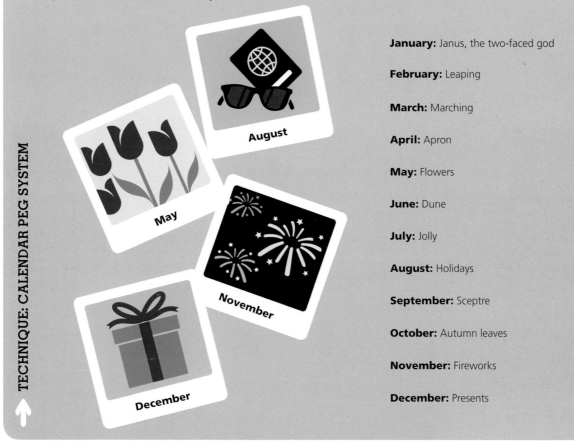

August

May

November

December

**TECHNIQUE: CALENDAR PEG SYSTEM**

**January:** Janus, the two-faced god

**February:** Leaping

**March:** Marching

**April:** Apron

**May:** Flowers

**June:** Dune

**July:** Jolly

**August:** Holidays

**September:** Sceptre

**October:** Autumn leaves

**November:** Fireworks

**December:** Presents

**TIP**

Making your memory cues concrete and visible is a time-honoured memory-boosting stratagem. Whether you use a traditional knot in a piece of string or a sticky note on the fridge, or whether you can come up with more creative options, aide mémoires kept in a visible place can help you circumvent memory problems.

## 6 CALENDAR PEG PRACTICE

Let's try out the calendar peg system – use it to memorize these six important events. When you're done, cover them up, name five ice-cream flavours, then see if you can recall them.

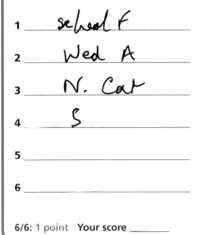

1 _school F_

2 _Wed A_

3 _N. Cat_

4 _S_

5 _____

6 _____

6/6: 1 point   Your score _____

**February**
feed neighbour's cat

**March**
school fête

**May**
wedding anniversary

**September**
back to school

**October**
holiday to France

**November**
international football match

## 7 DIARY DRAWER

Using the calendar peg system, can you turn these tasks and dates into memorable visual associations? Read the list then sketch simple but striking visual links in the diary. Cover the drawings, then recall the visualizations in order to remember during which month each task or event will take place.

End of season sale: **April**
House insurance renewal: **July**
Car service: **August**
Plant daffodil bulbs: **October**

August

July

October

April

4/4: 1 point   Your score _____

## 8 BIRTHDAY BIBLE

It's always handy if someone's birthday falls on a memorable date. For example, if Aunt Flora's birthday is on October 31, which is Halloween in many English-speaking countries, you can visualize a Jack o'lantern, which is symbolic of Halloween, as the face of a flower, to symbolize Flora. By thinking of some striking visuals to help you, practise memorizing these fake relatives' birthdays. Study them for 2 minutes, then cover and answer the questions.

Cousin Cleo's birthday is **4th July,** American Independence Day

Cousin Oliver's birthday is **11th November**, aka Remembrance Day, Armistice Day or Veteran's Day

Uncle Paul's birthday is **25th December**, Christmas Day

1 On which date is **Uncle Paul's** birthday?
2 Whose birthday is on **4th July**?
3 On which date is **cousin Oliver's** birthday?

1 _____

2 _____

3 _____

3/3: 1 point   Your score _____

## 9 BIRTHDAY BRAINIAC

A more generally applicable system for remembering the day as well as the month is to combine a calendar peg system with a number peg system.

For example, you always forget your niece Belle's birthday is **3rd May**.
Your calendar peg for May is a daffodil, so you could visualize Belle holding a daffodil.
Your rhyming number peg for 3 is sea, so you could visualize Belle floating in a boat on the sea.
To combine the two pegs, you could visualize Belle holding a daffodil while floating in a boat on the sea.

Use pegs of your own devising to memorize these birthdays. Then cover them up, recite your phone number backwards, and see if you can recall whose birthday is on which date.

Niece Belle: **3rd May**
Cousin Willy: **13th August**
Aunt Micha: **8th March**
Cousin Yoko: **25th April**
Nephew Sayed: **27th November**

1 _____

2 _____

3 _____

4 _____

5 _____

5/5: 1 point   Your score _____

## 10 ANNIVERSARY ACE

Birthdays aren't the only important biographical information you can memorize with a calendar/ number peg system combination. Use your personalized system to practise memorizing a few anniversaries of the sort that could really keep you out of trouble. Visualize the ones below for 2 minutes, then cover and test your recall after 5 minutes.

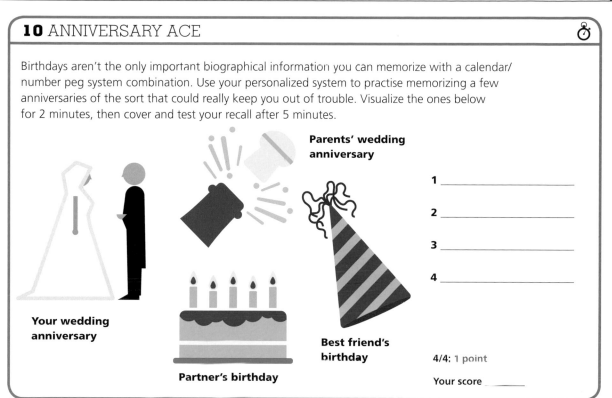

**Parents' wedding anniversary**

**Your wedding anniversary**

**Partner's birthday**

**Best friend's birthday**

1 _____

2 _____

3 _____

4 _____

4/4: 1 point

Your score _____

## 11 RETURN DATES

You've borrowed and renewed six books from the library, each due back on a different date. Can you remember the return dates by combining the calendar peg and number peg systems? Memorize, cover, and list eight Asian countries, then write down the due dates.

The Lost World: **10th January**
Around the World in 80 Days: **4th February**
The Hound of the Baskervilles: **6th April**
Treasure Island: **1st August**
Last of the Mohicans: **2nd September**
Frankenstein: **8th November**

return by
**10th January**

1 _____

2 _____

3 _____

4 _____

5 _____

6 _____

6/6: 1 point   Your score _____

## 12 GET KNOTTED

Another type of long-term memory is procedural memory – memory for "how" as opposed to memory for "what". When you learn a skill or routine, from learning to ride a bike to flying an aeroplane, you are creating long-term procedural memories. A good way to give your procedural memory a workout is to practise a useful or entertaining skill, such as tying a knot. Find two bits of string or rope, each at least 30cm (12in) long, and follow the simple instructions on the right to make a double fisherman's knot (a useful knot for tying two ropes together). Practise the knot six or seven times, and then come back a day later and try out the knot again. How did you get on?

**Score 1 point if you tied the knot correctly**

**Your score** _____

**1** Lie the ends of the two ropes together.

**2** With each rope, make two turns around both ropes, back in the direction of the rest of the rope.

**3** Pass the end through the loops and pull each end tight. You should end up with two "x" shapes.

## 13 KNOT KNOW-HOW

Using your procedural memory not only gives your brain a workout, but also teaches you useful practical skills. For instance, see if you can learn how to tie the knot known as a round turn and two half hitches, useful for tying a rope to a bar or ring. Follow the steps below, practise five or six times, then come back tomorrow and see how many steps you can recall. You can use rope or string.

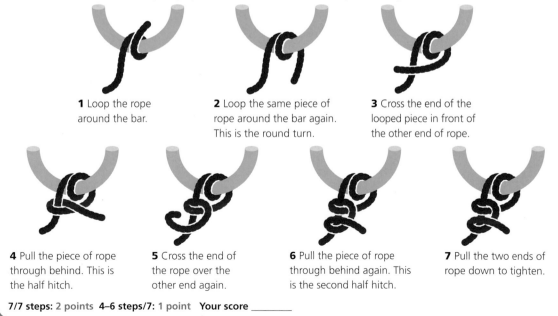

**1** Loop the rope around the bar.

**2** Loop the same piece of rope around the bar again. This is the round turn.

**3** Cross the end of the looped piece in front of the other end of rope.

**4** Pull the piece of rope through behind. This is the half hitch.

**5** Cross the end of the rope over the other end again.

**6** Pull the piece of rope through behind again. This is the second half hitch.

**7** Pull the two ends of rope down to tighten.

**7/7 steps: 2 points  4–6 steps/7: 1 point  Your score** _____

## 14 PICK UP A PENGUIN

Keep on working your procedural memory by learning to make this origami penguin. Take a square of paper and colour in one side (this is so the sides are clearly different). Start with the white side down and follow the instructions below. Practise with five squares of paper, then score yourself on how many folds you can remember.

**1** Turn the paper and fold in half to make a triangle.

**2** Fold a small top edge over. Repeat on the other side.

**3** With the sides still folded, open the paper out.

**4** Fold a small bottom piece inwards.

**5** Fold a small top piece behind to form the "head".

**6** Fold the paper in half.

**7** Push the head upwards.

6–7 folds: 2 points
4–5 folds: 1 point

**Your score** _____

## 15 ACE OF CUPS

Try this slightly more complex origami challenge – making a simple cup out of paper. Follow the visual instructions below and practise it five times, then score yourself on how many folds you can remember.

**1** Turn the paper so it's a rhombus shape. Fold in half.

**2** Fold a small triangle inwards, so it meets the edge.

**3** Fold a small triangle on the opposite side, so it aligns with the edge.

**4** Fold the first top triangle inwards.

**5** Fold the second top triangle behind.

**6** Pull the top two triangles, so the cup opens.

5–6 folds: 3 points
3–4 folds: 2 points
1–2 folds: 1 point

**Your score** _____

---

Your score    **/40**    **30–40 GOLD**

You have an excellent LTM for details big and small. Consider putting your gifts to good use by putting down your biographical memories on paper.

**10–29 SILVER**

Your LTM is average. Work through the chapter again in a few days: you may find that your memory has been stimulated in the interval and you can remember more.

**0–9 BRONZE**

There are some big spaces in your LTM and you should work on improving your encoding in the future. You can also fill in the blank spaces through exercises that stimulate biographical memories.

 Turn to page 178 for the Challenge

## CHAPTER 6

# PIN IN A HAYSTACK

## PINS AND PASSWORDS

# Pin in a haystack

Remembering many passwords and PINs can be tricky, especially as the guidelines governing their creation become ever more constrictive. This chapter will help you to create and recall secure and memorable passwords and provide tips for recalling PINs.

## QUESTIONNAIRE
Use this quick quiz to work out whether you're a security nightmare or a password paragon.

**1** Can you usually remember all your passwords, or do you have them written down?

**Remember/Written down
[score 1 point for "Remember"]**

**2** Do you frequently get locked out of your bank/email/shopping accounts?

**Frequently/Rarely
[score 1 point for "Rarely"]**

**3** Is your browser set to remember your passwords automatically?

**Yes/No
[score 1 point for "No"]**

**4** Have you left any of your passwords/PINs unchanged from the "password" or "1234" format in which they were initially given to you?

**Yes/No [score 1 point for "No"]**

**5** Have you used your own or a family member's name, your date of birth, a pet's name, or your home address for any of your passwords or PINs?

**Yes/No [score 1 point for "No"]**

**6** Do you have any sort of system for remembering different PINs and passwords, or do you just hope for the best?

**System/Hope for the best
[score 1 point for "System"]**

### How did you score?
**0–2:** Your memory for PINs and passwords is buckling under the weight of its daily demands, and you're cutting corners and compromising security as a result. The exercises in this chapter should help you to devise better and more memorable passwords.

**3–4:** You struggle to remember all your PINs and passwords, but the tips and techniques in this chapter should help you to improve.

**5–6:** You scored highly, but do you follow good practice on security as well as having a good memory for PINs and passwords? This chapter will help you cover all bases.

## 1 NAMES AND DATES

A useful source of personal information that combines letters and numbers is birthdays. Try putting together the first few letters of a relative or friend's name with their birth dates (don't use your own). For example, John Smith 15 February 1956 might become JoSm15Feb1956, or maybe 1956Jo15SmFeb. Practise on some of your relatives on a separate piece of paper.

| Relative | Name | Birth date |
|---|---|---|
| Father | _____ | _____ |
| Mother | _____ | _____ |
| Grandfather | _____ | _____ |
| Grandmother | _____ | _____ |
| Sibling | _____ | _____ |

## 2 LEETSPEAK

Leet derives from a computer user's "elite" status when accessing a software programme. Leetspeak became an online alphabet used by cybergeeks, in which the letters of the alphabet are replaced with symbols. This is a good system for creating a secure password. Using this table of leet substitutions, can you encode the five passwords?

**A** GOBULLDOGS  _____

**B** XYLOPHONE  _____

**C** BIRTHDAY  _____

**D** CALORIES  _____

**E** WHITEHOUSE  _____

| A @ | B \|3 | C ( | D \|) | E **3** | F \|= |
|---|---|---|---|---|---|
| G **9** | H **#** | I **!** | J _\| | K **1<** | L **1** |
| M **IVI** | N **IVI** | O ***** | P **IO** | Q **O_** | R **\|2** |
| S **$** | T **7** | U **L\|** | V **V** | W **VV** | X **%** |
| Y **´/,** | Z **2** | | | | |

Answers on page 180

**5/5: 1 point  Your score** _____

**TIP**

If you need help remembering a password, do not write down the password itself. Write a prompt or question, based on something personal, which will make sense to you but not to a thief. For example, if your password is based on something to do with a relative, use a private family nickname to remind you of the identity of the person.

## 3 STACKED UP

A clever trick that transforms your keyboard into a code machine is to use the column of letters under each number. For example, on the keyboard below, letters Q, A, and Z are below the number 1 key, while below the 6 are Y, H, and N (keyboards can differ so make sure you base your system on one that you use all the time). You can use this as the basis for a secure password by remembering a short number sequence, such as an important year, and typing all the letters under each number. For example, using the keyboard below, 1980 would be qazol.ik,p;/ Practise on these numbers.

| Numbers | Password |
|---|---|
| **A** 4046 | _____ |
| **B** 1979 | _____ |
| **C** 2005 | _____ |
| **D** 8238 | _____ |

**Answers on page 180**
**Score 4/4: 1 point   Your score** _____

## 4 BASE SYSTEM

Your passwords may be individually memorable, but how can you remember which one goes with which website or account? One way of doing so is to create a secure base password that you can use across multiple sites. Your base password is then individually tailored to each website or account, so you don't run the security risk of using the same password multiple times. The aim of this system is that you have to remember only your base password. The sites themselves then supply the key extra piece of information.

For your base password, make an acronym of something memorable, such as your favourite book, film title, or a line from a poem. For example, the phrase "Four And Twenty Blackbirds Baked In A Pie" becomes "4A20BBIAP". Practise creating a base password on the following:

**A** All For One And One For All          _____

**B** I Am 16 Going On 17          _____

**C** Three Blind Mice, See How They Run          _____

**D** Around The World In 80 Days          _____

**Answers on page 180**
**Score 4/4: 1 point   Your score** _____

## 5 SYSTEM ADDICT

If your base password does not contain any numbers, then it is a good idea to incorporate some. This will make your base much more secure. One easy and memorable way to do this is to precede the password with the number of words in the acronym. For example *Tyger, Tyger, Burning Bright, In The Forests Of The Night* becomes 10TTBBITFOTN. Practise creating memorable but secure base passwords with these examples.

**Full length**                    **Base password**

**A** The Unbearable Lightness Of Being          _____

**B** You Can't Always Get What You Want  _____

**C** To Kill A Mockingbird                 _____

**D** Red Sky At Night, Shepherd's Delight  _____

**Answers on page 181**

**4/4: 1 point  Your score** _____

## 6 BESPOKE PASSWORDS

Now practise modifying your base password to link it to the website for which it is used. A simple way to tailor the base password is to add three letters or numbers to it from the site or account name. For example, if your base password is 10TTBBITFOTN and the site is called www.moneybank.com, your site specific password could become mon10TTBBITFOTN. Using the same base, create passwords for these example sites:

**Site**                    **Bespoke password**

**A** www.green.com          _____

**B** www.evensquare.com   _____

**C** www.y3ksounds.org     _____

**D** www.legalbet.com      _____

**Answers on page 181**

**Score 4/4: 1 point  Your score** _____

## 7 CONSONANT SWAP

Another way to tailor your base password to each site is to substitute letters from the site name into your base, according to a preset rule. For example, you might have a rule that says "swap vowels in the site name with consonants in your base (as far as the number of letters will allow)". So for the website www.oakdoor.com and the base 10TTBBITFOTN you would swap the O for T, A for T, O for B, and O for B. Your password would become 10OAOOITFOTN. Practise using this rule with the same base and the example sites:

| Site | Bespoke password |
|------|------------------|
| **A** www.green.co.uk | _____ |
| **B** www.evensquare.com | _____ |
| **C** www.y3ksounds.org | _____ |
| **D** www.legalbet.com | _____ |

Answers on page 181

**Score 4/4: 1 point   Your score** _____

## 8 MADE TO MEASURE

You can make your base password even more secure and still tailor it to a website by changing it according to a characteristic of the site name. For instance, as well as adding the first letters of the site name you could also change the length of the base, so your password has an equal number of letters from both the website and the base. For example, suppose your base password is 10TTBBITFOTN and the website is oakdoor. You could take the first four letters of oakdoor and match it with the first four characters of your base to get the password oakd10TT. Using 10TTBBITFOTN as your base, tailor passwords for these example sites.

| Site | Bespoke password |
|------|------------------|
| **A** www.green.com | _____ |
| **B** www.evensquare.com | _____ |
| **C** www.y3ksounds.org | _____ |
| **D** www.legalbet.com | _____ |

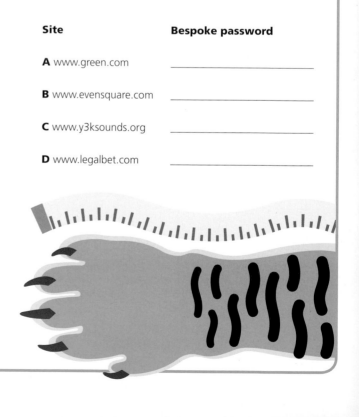

Answers on page 181

**Score 4/4: 1 point   Your score** _____

# 9 PASSWORD CREATION

Using your preferred system(s) from the password exercises you've just completed, create your own secure passwords for each of the eight holiday-related websites below. Try to remember these passwords, as you will be tested on them later in the chapter.

www.bank.com _____

www.willneedcarhire.com _____

www.bookonbeach.com _____

www.somewheretostay.com _____

www.moreclothes.com _____

www.bookwithus.com _____

www.flycheaply.com _____

www.mustbuyinsurance.com _____

## 10 PIN PRACTICE

Personal Identification Numbers (PINs) are only four digits long, but hard to remember when you have half a dozen of them jostling for space in your head. To set a baseline for your ability to remember PINs, try committing these four to memory, then cover them and come back at least an hour later to test your recall.

6012 _____

5585 _____

1003 _____

9174 _____

**Score 4/4: 1 point   Your score** _____

## 11 UP STACKED

The number stack system (see page 86) works in reverse to help you remember PINs. Each number in a four-digit PIN gives at least one corresponding letter option. Use these to then make a word or memorable acrostic. For example, if your PIN is 6546, you could choose the letters H, T, F, and N to come up with the acrostic Hard To Forget Now. If you have access to a keyboard, all you have to do is remember the acrostic. Using the keyboard below, work out these PINs from their acrostics, within 1 minute.

| **Acrostic** | **PIN** |
| --- | --- |
| **A** Too Easy To Remember | _____ |
| **B** I Love Purple Shoes | _____ |
| **C** North South East West | _____ |
| **D** Once Upon A Time | _____ |

**Answers on page 181**
**Score 4/4 within 1 minute: 1 point   Your score** _____

## 12 FOUR-WORD DECODER

Linking your PIN to a visual sentence is a good way of recalling the numbers. Use the numbers in a PIN to dictate the length of the words in a four-word sentence. For example, 3734 would yield a sentence with words three letters, seven letters, three letters, and four letters long respectively. For example, "bad manners are rude". Based on the number of letters in the words in the phrases below, can you decode them into PINs? Cover the PINs, wait 30 minutes, and see if you can write them down on a separate piece of paper.

| Four-word sentence | PIN |
|---|---|
| Dancing down the road | _____ |
| Happy hippos gamble gladly | _____ |
| Little ants attacked me | _____ |
| Men wearing enormous pants | _____ |
| Into the unknown outside | _____ |

**Score 5/5: 1 point   Your score** _____

## 13 FOUR-WORD KEYS

Now practise generating your own four-word sentences. For each of the three PINs below, can you devise a four-word mnemonic? When you have done so, come back to the exercise after an hour and, with the PINs and mnemonics covered up, see if you can recall the PINs using your mnemonics, on a separate piece of paper.

| PIN | Four-word sentence |
|---|---|
| 5324 | _____ |
| | _____ |
| 8437 | _____ |
| | _____ |
| 6244 | _____ |
| | _____ |

**Score 3/3: 1 point   Your score** _____

**TIP**

Some of the more realistic cyber-security experts concede that if it's a choice between people using unsafe passwords or writing something down, the latter may be more secure. With a secret note you can physically control access to it as well as physically concealing it, and you are more likely to be able to tell if security has been compromised. So consider writing down at least a cryptic hint for self-reminder purposes.

## 14 LETTER PAIRS

A simple mnemonic technique for PINs is to treat the numbers as code for a sequence of letters. Let the first 10 letters of the alphabet correspond to the numbers 0–9 and translate your PIN into a four-letter sequence: A would be 0, B would be 1 and so on. If you treat these four numbers as two pairs of letters and use the pairs as the initials of famous people, you have a base for a memorable visualization. For example, if your PIN is 1631, the corresponding letter pairs will be B (1) G (6) and D (3) B (1), which could suggest the famous names Bee Gees and David Beckham. Come up with a visualization to combine the two names and you have a mnemonic for your PIN. Try the technique on these PINs, using a separate piece of paper if necessary.

| PIN | Letters | Famous names | Visualization |
|-----|---------|--------------|---------------|
| 4407 | | | |
| 6383 | | | |
| 3251 | | | |

## 15 LETTER PAIRS PLUS

Using only the first 10 letters of the alphabet is restrictive. To use the full range for the same initials-generating technique, refer to a table such as this:

| 0 | 1 | 2 | 3 | 4 | 5 | 6 | 7 | 8 | 9 |
|---|---|---|---|---|---|---|---|---|---|
| A | B | C | D | E | F | G | H | I | J |
| K | L | M | N | O | P | Q | R | S | T |
| U | V | W | X | Y | Z | | | | |

Use the table to work out the PINs represented by these famous pairs. Then cover the PINs and table and try to recall the PINs 5 minutes later.

| Names | Initials | Corresponding PIN |
|-------|----------|-------------------|
| **A** Arnold Schwarzenegger and The Pink Panther | | |
| **B** Tom Cruise and John Travolta | | |
| **C** Woody Allen and Barack Obama | | |
| **D** Elvis Presley and Mahatma Gandhi | | |

**Answers on page 181**
**Score 4/4: 1 point   Your score _____**

## 16 WORD PINS

For some PINs, the number–letter system will yield letter sequences that are words or are close to words: for example, 5748 converts to PRES, which is short for "president". In such cases you will only need to remember a single word. Using the chart of number–letter correspondences in exercise 15, turn these PINs into words, commit them to memory, and then cover the list. Write down eight American actors, then see if you can remember the words and the numbers to which they correspond.

| PIN | Word | PIN recall |
|---|---|---|
| 8203 | | |
| 3429 | | |
| 1011 | | |
| 0836 | | |
| 4668 | | |

## 17 PIN PUNS

Some numbers have ready-made associations; for example, 4 is the number of sides in a square. Use common associations like this as the basis for creating memorable visualizations, and if possible make them humorous. For example, 3375 might suggest two triangles (3 being the number of sides of a triangle) and a grandfather (75 could be the age of your grandfather when you were born). This could suggest the image of a grandfather trying to ride a bicycle with two triangular wheels. Come up with memorable visuals for these PINs, then try to recall them after 30 minutes.

| PIN | Visualization |
|---|---|
| 7213 | |
| 9249 | |
| 1001 | |
| 1865 | |

4/4: 1 point   **Your score** _____

93

## 18 NUMBER RHYMES

You can use rhymes to help remember your PINs. Write down memorable rhyming words for numbers 0–9. Once you've come up with a list of rhyming words, use them to create a sentence with a memorable visualization for your PINs. For example, if your PIN is 8513, you could create the visual sentence: a great (8) drive (5) in the sun (1) to a tree (3). See if you can use your rhyming words to think of visualizations for the PINs below. Now cover the PINs and after 30 minutes see if you can recall the PINs through the visualizations.

*6036*

| | **Visualization** | **Pin recall** |
|---|---|---|
| 6036 | _____ | _____ |
| 1523 | _____ | _____ |
| 8470 | _____ | _____ |
| 9845 | _____ | _____ |

**Score 1 point** for each PIN you remember **Your score** _____

## 19 THIS OLD MAN

Another system for turning numbers into memorable images is based on nursery rhymes, such as *This Old Man,* which rhymes numbers with words. For example, two and shoe, three and knee. You can then use these words to construct a visualization. On the right are the rhymes from *This Old Man*, plus an extra one for zero.

Using the rhymes for *This Old Man*, can you decode these sentences into their corresponding PINs?

**A** Use shoes and thumbs to push open the gate to heaven     **PIN** _____

**B** Superhero uses a stick to open door to reveal a beehive     **PIN** _____

**C** Shoes that are best for your spine and knees are by the door     **PIN** _____

| Number | Rhyme |
|---|---|
| 1 | thumb |
| 2 | shoe |
| 3 | knee |
| 4 | door |
| 5 | hive |
| 6 | sticks |
| 7 | heaven |
| 8 | gate |
| 9 | spine |
| 0 | hero |

**Answers on page 181    3/3: 1 point   Your score** _____

# 20 PASSWORD RECALL

Your week of sun and sand – all booked and arranged online – turns into an eventful trip. At an internet café, you need to access the various sites you used to arrange the holiday, but can you remember all the passwords you created on page 89?

You want to book another excursion through the same company. Recall your password to book again.

www.bookwithus.com

It's time to check in for the flight home. What is your password for the airline website?

www.flycheaply.com

The hotel cannot find your booking. Log on to your account to find the booking confirmation.

www.somewheretostay.com

You've finished all your books. Can you access the online bookstore to download more?

www.bookonbeach.com

You need to make a claim on your travel insurance. Log on to your account to find your policy.

www.mustbuyinsurance.com

Your wallet has been stolen. Can you recall your password for your bank to transfer emergency funds?

www.bank.com

You've been given a small car, when you booked a large family car. Log on to the car rental website to sort it out.

www.willneedcarhire.com

The online department store sent you the wrong clothing items. Log on to the site to request a return.

www.moreclothes.com

**Score 1 point for each password you remembered   Your score _____**

---

Your score   **/35**

**30–35 GOLD**
Your memory for passwords and PINs is impressive – keep practising your memorization techniques to make them perfect.

**20–29 SILVER**
Your memory for passwords and PINs is fair, but could improve. Revisit the methods of memorization in this chapter and keep practising them.

**0–19 BRONZE**
PINs and passwords pose a significant challenge to your memory abilities. Go back and work through the chapter again.

⭐ Turn to page 178 for the Challenge.

CHAPTER 7
# REVISION EXPRESS
RECALL OF FACTS

# Revision express

Any memory that can be recalled after a minute has been stored in your long-term memory. A subcategory of long-term memory is semantic memory, which is knowledge-based and not related to personal, or emotional, experiences. Facts, rules, meanings, and any general knowledge you have learnt are all stored, and retrieved, from your semantic memory.

## QUESTIONNAIRE

Are you a quiz champion and exam expert or a forgetful fumbler of facts? Use this quick quiz to see how your semantic memory shapes up in your everyday life.

**1** If you were taking part in a charity quiz night, do you think you would be a help or a hindrance?

**Help/Hindrance**
[score 1 point for "Help"]

**2** Would you prefer to be academically assessed with exams or coursework?

**Exams/Coursework**
[score 1 point for "Exams"]

**3** When you play a trivia game, are you usually in the winning or losing team?

**Winning/Losing**
[score 1 point for "Winning"]

**4** At an amusement arcade you notice a general knowledge quiz machine that offers big prizes, but costs little to play. Would you take it on?

**Take it on/Walk on by**
[score 1 point for "Take it on"]

**5** When you watch quiz shows on TV, do you find yourself shouting out the answers to the contestants?

**Often/Sometimes**
[score 1 point for "Often"]

**6** A child asks you to explain how a rainbow is made – how accurate is your answer?

**Accurate/Confused**
[score 1 point for "Accurate"]

### How did you score?

**0–2:** Your knowledge base is lacking – you probably need to work on boosting both your encoding and retrieval of semantic memory.

**3–4:** Your semantic memory is average. The exercises and challenges in this chapter should help you to reach the top of the class.

**5–6:** You're a bit of a boffin, but you can always do better. The exercises in this chapter should help hone your mental edge.

## 1 QUIZ MASTER

A good way to get a baseline of your semantic memory is to test your general knowledge. See how you score in this test.

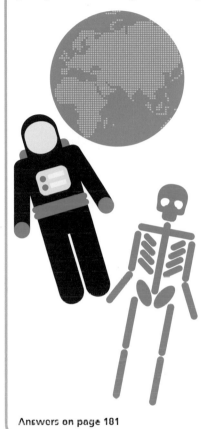

**1** What is the second most populous nation on Earth?

**2** Who composed the Moonlight Sonata?

**3** Can you name all the world's oceans?

**4** Complete Sir Isaac Newton's famous third law of motion: "For every action..."

**5** In which country was the compass invented?

**6** What year was the Russian Revolution?

**7** Who was the second man on the Moon?

**8** What is the longest bone in the body?

**9** Which national team won the first football World Cup?

**10** Which individual has won the most oscars?

1 _____

2 _____

3 _____

4 _____

5 _____

6 _____

7 _____

8 _____

9 _____

10 _____

Answers on page 181

**Score 1 point for each correct answer**

**Your score** _____

## 2 SPOT THE LINK

There are more (and arguably better) ways to test knowledge than a straightforward general knowledge quiz. For instance, putting your knowledge to work in a test such as this: can you work out what these countries have in common?

**Luxembourg**

**San Marino**

**Bolivia**

**Nepal**

**Paraguay**

**Answer**_____

Answer on page 181

**Score 3 points for a correct answer**
**Your score** _____

A mnemonic is a device that aids memorization. An acrostic is one example of a mnemonic. Here, a list of facts to be memorized is replaced with a more memorable list of words with the same initial letter. Acrostics can be very helpful when you need to remember facts in a particular order. Here is an example of an acrostic to help you remember the order of the planets from the Sun. When prompted, your acrostic should spring to mind, and can then be converted back into the fact.

| Fact | Acrostic | Prompt |
|---|---|---|
| Order of the planets from the Sun (Mercury, Venus, Earth, Mars, Jupiter, Saturn, Uranus, Neptune) | My Very Easy Method: Just Sit Up Nights | Name the planets in order |

## 3 MORE MNEMONIC ACROSTICS

Try out some more acrostics for a rapid-learning technique. See if you can devise memorable acrostics to help you recall these three facts, then give yourself 30 seconds to learn them. Cover and use the prompt to test your recall after waiting 5 minutes.

| Fact | Acrostic | Prompt | Fact recall |
|---|---|---|---|
| Attributes of living things in biology (Nutrition, Irritability, Movement, Growth, Respiration, Reproduction, Excretion) | _____ _____ | List the attributes of living things in biology | _____ _____ |
| Order in which notes fall on the treble clef (EGBDF) | _____ _____ | List the notes of the treble clef in order | _____ |
| How to spell "rhythm" | _____ _____ | Spell the word that means the regular beat of a piece of music | _____ |

**3/3: Score 1 point  Your score** _____

Mnemonics can help you to commit small pieces of information to memory, but a large amount of information needs a more comprehensive solution. The first step in boosting memory for semantic knowledge is to improve encoding – facts become more memorable when they are learned in context, rather than in isolation. In other words, learning additional information can make the central data easier to remember.

On the right is an isolated fact, then a different fact accompanied by some background information. Read both, then wait 20 minutes before returning and testing for recall (with the information covered up). It should be easier to remember the fact with extra information.

**Isolated fact**
Chemical symbol for silver: Ag

**Fact with background information**
Chemical symbol for sodium: Na.
Na derives from natron, the Egyptian word for salt, because sodium is one of the elements that makes up salt (sodium chloride).
The Egyptians used natron to dry out and preserve corpses as part of the mummification process.

# 4 BACKGROUND CHECK PRACTICE

Read the following facts and concentrate carefully on their background information to help you to encode them. Now cover the facts and the background information, wait 5 minutes, then see if you can answer the questions below.

### The newton is the unit for force
The unit for force is named after physicist Sir Issac Newton, whose third law of motion stated that for every force acting in one direction, there is an equal force acting in the opposite direction.

### The capital of the Republic of Congo is Brazzaville
Brazzaville is named after the Italian-French explorer Pierre Savorgnan de Brazza. Brazza's explorations along the Congo River helped France establish its colony known as French Congo.

### Antonin Dvorák was a Czech composer
Dvorák was born in Bohemia, then part of the Austro-Hungarian Empire. He studied at the Organ School in Prague.

### Quiz questions

**1** What is the capital of the Republic of Congo? _____

**2** What is the unit for force? _____

**3** What nationality was Dvorák? _____

**Score 1 point for each correct answer   Your score _____**

**TECHNIQUE: TOPLINE**

One of the keys to better revision is smarter revision. Don't try to commit whole chunks of text to memory; work through the text and identify the topline facts and key words – these can become the bullet points that you should try to commit to memory. For example, on the right is a small extract about bats from an encyclopaedia of animals.

You could pick out the following bullet points from it:
• **Bats are the only mammals that can fly, rather than glide.**
• **The wing membrane is called the patagium.**

Bats are the only mammals that possess true, flapping wings and the ability to fly (as opposed to colugos, for example, which glide). Bats' wing membrane (the patagium), an extension of the skin of the back and belly, provides a high degree of manoeuvrability in flight.

## **5** TOPLINE PRACTICE

Here is the rest of the passage on bats from the encyclopaedia. Can you highlight five topline facts within the passage, then recall them below after 30 minutes.

1 _____
_____

2 _____
_____

3 _____
_____

4 _____
_____

5 _____
_____

How many facts did you recall?
5/5: score 2 points
3–4/5: score 1 point

Your score _____

Bats' wingspans range from over 1.5m (5ft) in the large flying fox to as little as 15cm (6in) in the hog-nosed bat. Over half the species echolocate to capture prey and to navigate at night. Chiropetra is a huge order that comprises nearly a quarter of all mammal species and is exceeded only by rodents in terms of species numbers. Bats are common in tropical and temperate habitats worldwide, but are not found in environments that are too cold to support a source of food, such as the polar regions. When used in flight, echolocation makes bats formidable hunters. Sounds ("clicks") are produced in the larynx, emitted through the nose or mouth, and directed or focused by the nose leaf (if present). Once the clicks have reflected off an object, the returning echo is picked up via the bat's sensitive ears. The time it takes to receive the echo reveals the size and location of anything in the bat's path.

A popular visual tool for boosting learning and revision, that can help with both encoding and retrieval, is a Mind Web. This is a diagram showing information, or just single words, in boxes or circles, and associated words or concepts joined to them and to other information by lines, to give a branching, tree-like structure radiating out from the centre. The addition of graphics adds a visual element to the Mind Web, which can aid semantic memorization. Below is a simple example based around a play you might be studying. Can you draw a Mind Web for a topic of your choice?

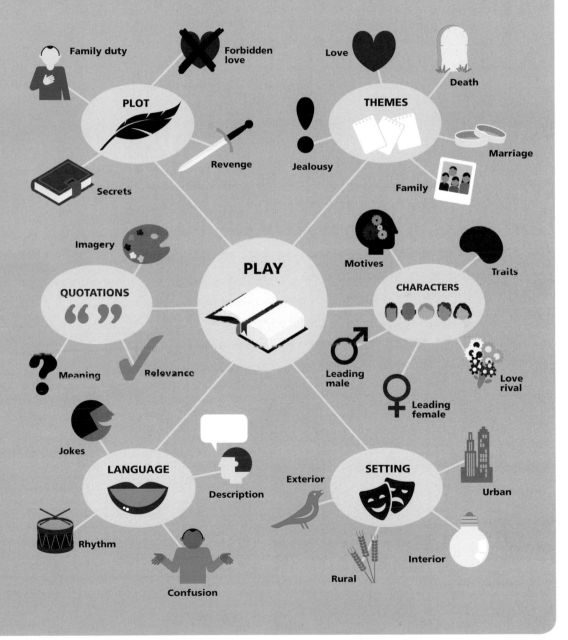

TECHNIQUE: MENTAL MAPPING

Visualization can help you learn and remember all sorts of facts. For instance, if you are 1.8m (6ft) tall, you could remember that the longest boa constrictor ever found was 5.4m (18ft) long, by picturing three of you alongside it end to end. Try to think of a visualization for the facts you need to learn and see if you find them easier to recall.

**TIP**

Repeating an act of memorization five times is believed to fix a fact irrevocably in your LTM. Whether or not this is true, it certainly helps to review pieces of information at regular intervals – frequently at first, then at longer intervals. For instance, review first after an hour, then after a day, then after a week.

# 6 SCIENCE FICTION PRACTICE

Practise some visual associations on these science facts, then see if you can answer the questions 10 minutes later.

**Nitrogen** is the most common gas in the atmosphere.

The dinosaurs died out **65 million years ago**.

The nearest star to our Solar System is **Proxima Centauri**.

Almost 50% of human being's DNA is identical to that of a **banana**.

Rivers and lakes account for less than **0.007 per cent** of the Earth's water.

_____ is the most common gas in the atmosphere.

The dinosaurs died out _____

The nearest star to our Solar System is _____

What percentage of DNA do humans share with a banana? _____

Rivers and lakes account for less than _____ per cent of the Earth's water.

**Score 1 point for each fact you remembered**

**Your score** _____

Peg systems involve learning a memorable series, which can then form the basis of a sequence of visualizations (see pages 50, 62, and 76 for examples). The body makes a good basis for a peg system, if you learn its "numbering". Learn all the locations and you can memorize lists up to 15 items long – more if you wish to create further pegs. For example, if you needed to memorize the instruments in an orchestra, you could relate the first instrument on your list, say a violin, to the first body peg, in this example the head. So you could visualize the violin's resonances (the f-shaped airholes) as a moustache. Study the list of pegs below for as long as you need, then cover it and write down all the locations in order.

**TECHNIQUE: BODY PEG SYSTEM**

1 Head
2 Eyes
3 Nose
4 Ears
5 Mouth
6 Chin
7 Shoulder
8 Chest
9 Arm
10 Elbow
11 Hand
12 Fingertips
13 Stomach
14 Knee
15 Foot

# 7 BATTLE STATIONS

Try out the body peg system by learning this list of major battles of the Second World War. Link the first battle on the list to the first peg of the human body and form a visualization for each battle. Cover the list, name five species of trees, and see if you can reproduce it.

**1** Battle of Dunkirk

**2** Battle of the River Plate

**3** Battle of Britain

**4** Attack on Pearl Harbour

**5** The Battle of Moscow

**6** The Battle of Stalingrad

**7** The Fall of Singapore

**8** D-Day Landings

**9** The Battle of Arnhem

**10** The Battle of the Bulge

**11** The Battle of Berlin

**12** The Battle of Coral Sea

**13** The Battle of Midway

**14** The Battle of Guadalcanal

**15** The Battle of the Philippine Sea

1 _____
2 _____
3 _____
4 _____
5 _____
6 _____
7 _____
8 _____
9 _____
10 _____
11 _____
12 _____
13 _____
14 _____
15 _____

**Score 1 point for each battle you remembered**

**Your score** _____

## 8 FACTUAL STORIES

Another peg system that can work well for semantic knowledge is taking a familiar narrative and using the narrative's stages as pegs. You can then create visualizations between your list of facts to remember and the pegs. For instance, take the tale of The Hare and the Tortoise. You could peg events from Australian history to the stages of the story. Use the information below as the basis for a series of visualizations, then cover the first column and test for recall in 10 minutes.

| Australian history | Hare & Tortoise |
|---|---|
| First humans cross from Indonesia | Hare laughs at slow Tortoise |
| Evolution of Aboriginal culture | Tortoise challenges Hare |
| Introduction of dingo | Hare takes early lead |
| First European explorers sight Australia | Hare takes nap |
| Captain Cook visits Australia | Tortoise overtakes Hare |
| Establishment of Sydney colony | Hare wakes up |
| Circumnavigation of Australia | Tortoise wins race |

Score **1 point** for each event you remembered and **2 extra points** if they are in the correct order   Your score _____

1 _____

2 _____

3 _____

4 _____

5 _____

6 _____

7 _____

## 9 OPERATIC PROGRESS

Another type of peg system, related to the one above, is the journey system (see page 62), in which stages in a memorable journey are the pegs, and the items to remember are connected to those journey stages through visualizations. Can you commit to memory seven operas by Mozart using stages on a familiar journey such as your commute to work? Use the system to memorize them, then cover the list, write down the names of five rivers, and see if you can remember the operas in order.

**Don Giovanni**
**Così fan tutte**
**The Impresario**
**The Magic Flute**
**The Shepherd King**
**The Marriage of Figaro**
**Thamos, King of Egypt**

1 _____

2 _____

3 _____

4 _____

5 _____

6 _____

7 _____

Score **1 point** for each opera you remembered   Your score _____

## 10 POET'S CORNER

Use one of the techniques described in this chapter to memorize the list of famous 19th-century poets below. Once you've committed the list to memory, cover it up, wait 10 minutes, then see if you can name all the poets on the list.

**Emily Dickinson**
**Thomas Hardy**
**Walt Whitman**
**Wilfred Owen**
**Robert William Service**
**Harriet Beecher Stowe**
**Robert Graves**

1 _____    6 _____

2 _____    7 _____

3 _____

4 _____    Score **1 point** for each
                      poet you remembered

5 _____    Your score _____

## 11 MOBS AND GANGS

Now choose a different technique from the chapter and practise using it to memorize this list of collective nouns for animals. Once you've committed the list to memory, cover it up, list your five favourite books, and see if you can remember all the collective nouns.

**A gang of elks**         **A parliament of rooks**
**A murder of crows**      **An unkindness of ravens**
                           **A labour of moles**
                           **A pod of porpoises**
                           **A mob of kangaroos**

1 _____    6 _____

2 _____    7 _____

3 _____

4 _____    Score **1 point** for each
                      collective noun you
                      remembered

5 _____    Your score _____

---

Your score    **/75**     **60–75 GOLD**

You are a trivia sponge and excellent at learning new information. The tips and techniques in this chapter may help you to become even more effective.

**30–59 SILVER**

You find some topic areas tougher than others, and possibly some techniques more effective than others. Identify which techniques work best for you and stick with those.

**0–29 BRONZE**

You are struggling to learn/remember new facts. Have a look at the techniques in this chapter again: they might help improve your ability to encode and retrieve, preparing you for another assault on the exercises.

 Turn to page 179 for the Challenge.

## CHAPTER 8

# A HEAD FOR FIGURES

## BASIC NUMERACY

# A head for figures

This chapter looks at the simplest forms of numerical intelligence, from basic arithmetic and proportions to "real world" problems involving simple maths. Where possible, do the calculations in your head and use a calculator only where stated.

## QUESTIONNAIRE

Are you a human calculator or a calculating catastrophe? Take this quick quiz to see how your maths skills match up.

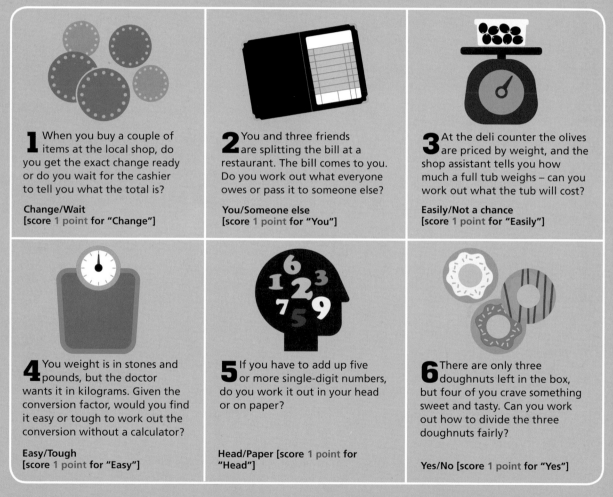

**1** When you buy a couple of items at the local shop, do you get the exact change ready or do you wait for the cashier to tell you what the total is?

**Change/Wait**
**[score 1 point for "Change"]**

**2** You and three friends are splitting the bill at a restaurant. The bill comes to you. Do you work out what everyone owes or pass it to someone else?

**You/Someone else**
**[score 1 point for "You"]**

**3** At the deli counter the olives are priced by weight, and the shop assistant tells you how much a full tub weighs – can you work out what the tub will cost?

**Easily/Not a chance**
**[score 1 point for "Easily"]**

**4** You weight is in stones and pounds, but the doctor wants it in kilograms. Given the conversion factor, would you find it easy or tough to work out the conversion without a calculator?

**Easy/Tough**
**[score 1 point for "Easy"]**

**5** If you have to add up five or more single-digit numbers, do you work it out in your head or on paper?

**Head/Paper [score 1 point for "Head"]**

**6** There are only three doughnuts left in the box, but four of you crave something sweet and tasty. Can you work out how to divide the three doughnuts fairly?

**Yes/No [score 1 point for "Yes"]**

### How did you score?

**0–2:** Basic numeracy is a problem, which can be frustrating in day-to-day life and could have serious consequences in areas such as personal finance and financial security. Working through this chapter will give your arithmetic skills a workout and should boost your confidence.

**3–4:** Your basic numerical reasoning skills are average, but there is plenty of room for improvement by giving your brain an arithmetical workout.

**5–6:** You are numerate, but how speedy are you when it comes to mental arithmetic? Hone your skills by seeing how fast you can blitz through these exercises.

## 1 ARITHMETIC 101

Working them out in your head, can you do these sums?

**A** 337 + 884 = _____ *1221*

**B** 7206 + 5997 = _____ *1 3203*

**C** 543 − 297 = _____ *840 246*

**D** 11,063 − 7789 = _____ *3274*

**E** 63 x 11 = _____ *693*

**F** 76 x 87 = _____

**G** 121 ÷ 11 = _____ *11*

**H** 91 ÷ 7 = _____ *13*

Answers on page 181
Score **1 point** for each correct answer
Your score _____

## 2 RAISING CHANGE

You are a cashier in a shop, but your till has broken. Work out the change due to each customer.

**Change due**

**A** The customer buys a pack of batteries (£5.85), and pays with a £10 note. _____ *4.15*

**B** The customer buys some lip balm (£2.11), apples (85p), and a postcard (99p), and pays with a £5 note. _____ *1.05*

**C** The customer buys a chocolate bar (85p), a bottle of water (£1.90), a newspaper (£2.31), and a magazine (£5.99), and pays with a £20 note. _____ *8.95*

**D** The customer buys a newspaper (£2.31), a pack of gum (99p), a packet of biscuits (£3.99), a bottle of wine (£10.86), and a lighter (£1.13), and pays with a £20 note and 30p in change. _____ *£1.10*

Answers on page 181
Score **1 point** for each correct answer
Your score _____

## 3 PAPERBACK PROBLEM

At the bookshop you find three books you want to buy. You only have £17.50 – which books can you afford and how much change will you receive?

**The Secret Lives of Aunts**

£7.99

£9.99

**Coffee and Cheese**

**Year of the Yak**

£8.99

**Answer** _____

Answer on page 181
Score **1 point** for a correct answer   Your score _____

## 4 CANDY CONUNDRUM

There are five jars of sweets behind the counter at the sweet shop, labelled with the price per sweet. You have 95 pence to spend. What is the maximum number of sweets you can get for your money?

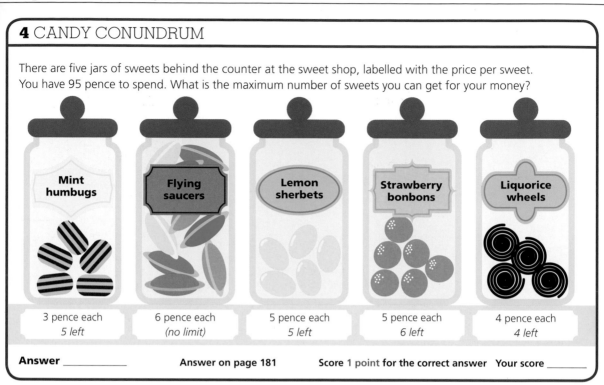

| Mint humbugs | Flying saucers | Lemon sherbets | Strawberry bonbons | Liquorice wheels |
|---|---|---|---|---|
| 3 pence each | 6 pence each | 5 pence each | 5 pence each | 4 pence each |
| *5 left* | *(no limit)* | *5 left* | *6 left* | *4 left* |

**Answer** _____          **Answer on page 181**          Score **1 point** for the correct answer   **Your score** _____

## 5 ARE YOU COORDINATED?

Graphs are a way of mapping out points and lines according to their coordinates in a two-dimensional space. If X is the horizontal axis and Y is the vertical axis, what are the coordinates of the points on this graph? Give the x axis coordinate first.

**A** _____

**B** _____

**C** _____

**D** _____

**E** _____

Answers on page 181
5/5: 1 point  Your score _____

## **6** GOLDEN BOOTY

The king has two chests in his treasure chamber – a wooden chest and a heavy-lidded steel chest. He moves a bag of 100 gold coins from the wooden chest to the steel chest. He now has three times as many coins in the steel chest than he has in the wooden one. He has 2,000 coins in total. How many coins were in each chest before he moved the bag?

**Answer** _____ 　　　**Answer on page 181** 　　　**Score 1 point for a correct answer　Your score** _____

## **7** WHICH IS BIGGER? I

Rank these fractions in order of size, from the biggest to the smallest:

¾

⅔

⅞

⁹⁄₁₆

⅖

⁵⁄₁₅

2　**1** _____

3　**2** _____

1　**3** _____

4　**4** _____

5　**5** _____

6　**6** _____

**Answer on page 181**
**6/6: 1 point　Your score** _____

## **8** WHICH IS BIGGER? II

Rank these fractions in order of size, from the biggest to the smallest:

⅝

¹⁵⁄₃₂

⅔

⁶⁄₁₀

⁹⁄₁₂

⁸⁄₁₅

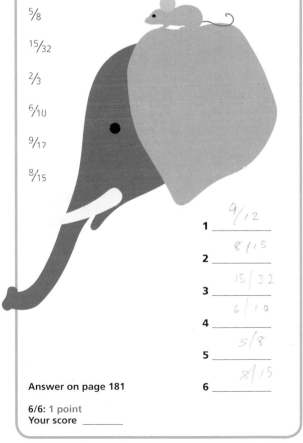

**1** ___9/12___

**2** ___8/15___

**3** ___15/32___

**4** ___6/10___

**5** ___5/8___

**6** ___8/15___

**Answer on page 181**

**6/6: 1 point**
**Your score** _____

## 9 DECIMALS VS FRACTIONS I

Rank these fractions and decimals in order of size, from the biggest to the smallest:

0.6        0.3

²/₃        0.8

¼          ²/₆

1  ___0.8___          4  ___¼___

2  ___2/3___          5  ___2/6___

3  ___0.3___          6  ___0.3___

Answer on page 181

**6/6: 1 point   Your score** _____

## 10 DECIMALS VS FRACTIONS II

Rank these fractions and decimals in order of size, from the biggest to the smallest:

0.275

²/₅

⁷/₃₂

¹¹/₂₁

0.5

0.333

11/21

1  ___0.5___

2  ___2/5___

3  _____

4  ___.333___

5  ___0.275___

6  ___7/32___

Answer on page 181

**6/6: 1 point**
**Your score** _____

## 11 SOCK PUZZLE

Derek has checked socks and spotty socks. For every six pairs of checked socks, he has nine pairs of spotty socks. If there are 50 pairs of socks in his sock drawer, how many pairs of checked socks does he have?

**Answer** _____

Answer on page 182        Score **1 point** for a correct answer   Your score _____

## 12 SLICE OF THE PIE

A pie chart is a graphical representation of proportions. Can you write as a fraction the proportions represented by each slice of these pie charts?

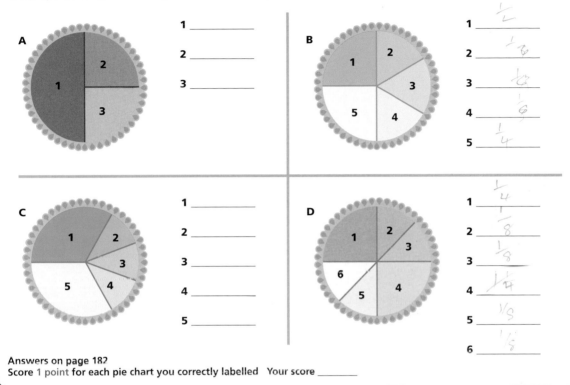

**A**

1 _____

2 _____

3 _____

**B**

1 $\frac{1}{2}$

2 $\frac{1}{8}$

3 $\frac{1}{8}$

4 $\frac{1}{6}$

5 $\frac{1}{4}$

**C**

1 _____

2 _____

3 _____

4 _____

5 _____

**D**

1 $\frac{1}{4}$

2 $\frac{1}{8}$

3 $\frac{1}{8}$

4 $\frac{1}{4}$

5 $\frac{1}{8}$

6 $\frac{1}{8}$

**Answers on page 182**
**Score 1 point** for each pie chart you correctly labelled   Your score _____

## 13 STAR STRUCK

Gazing out from the stage, you wonder what proportion of your audience are students on concessionary tickets. The theatre holds 160 people, but it is only three-quarters full, and 90 of the audience members are students. What percentage of the audience is students?

**Answer** _____

**Answer on page 182**
**Score 1 point** for a correct answer   Your score _____

## 14 LITTLE BROTHER

A woman tells you that the average age of her three sons is eight, but they are all under 10. What is the youngest any of them can be?

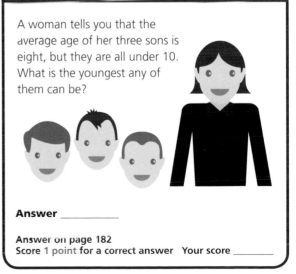

**Answer** _____

**Answer on page 182**
**Score 1 point** for a correct answer   Your score _____

b.0₀₀

## 15 CHEESE PLEASE

In the cheese shop the offerings are priced per kilogram.
Can you work out how much the following orders will cost?

**A** 200g Roquefort
750g Gruyère

*(handwritten: 3·10, 12·10)*

**B** 750g Edam
500g Roquefort
250g Brie

*(handwritten: 1·17, 7·75, 1·9?)*

**C** 250g Camembert
400g Roquefort
750g Gruyère
150g Edam

*(handwritten: 2·10, 6, 9, 2·30, 19·40)*

**Edam** £5.90/kg

**Brie** £7.70/kg

**Roquefort** £15.50/kg

**Camembert** £8.40/kg

**Gruyère** £12/kg

**Answers on page 182**
**Score 1 point** for each correct answer   Your score _____

## 16 HENRY'S CAT

Henry is four years older than his cat, but eight years ago Henry was twice as old as his cat. How old is Henry?

**Answer** _____

**Answer on page 182**
**Score 1 point** for a correct answer   Your score _____

## 17 BILL BRAINTEASER

Your currency has bank notes in the denominations 5, 10, and 20. Given the number of notes in your wallet and their total value, can you work out what is the lowest value note you could have in each case?

| Number of notes | Total value | Lowest value note |
|---|---|---|
| **A** 3 | 40 | 10 |
| **B** 4 | 40 | 5 |
| **C** 4 | 50 | 5 |
| **D** 5 | 60 | 10 |

**Answers on page 182**
**Score 1 point** for each correct answer   Your score _____

## 18 WHAT TIME IS IT? I

A series of sequential numbers are grouped together by a base. For example, our normal counting system is base 10; we count from 0 to 9 as single digits, and 10, which means "one 10" and "zero single units". (So the number 210 means "two 100s", "one 10", and "no single units"). In everyday life we use bases when talking about the time. Hours, for instance, are in base 12, and minutes and second are in base 60. Practise using base 12 here:

**A** In 17 hours it will be 2am, what time is it now?

**Answer** _____

**B** In 16 hours you will be eight hours late for your 9am appointment. What time is it now?

**Answer** _____

**C** Stockholm is seven hours behind Singapore. If it is 11am in Singapore, what time will it be in Stockholm 16 hours from now?

**Answer** _____

**D** Melbourne is 16 hours ahead of New York, which is five hours behind London. Eric leaves Melbourne at 4pm local time and flies to London. According to his watch, which is on New York time, he touches down at 1pm. How long was his flight and what is the local time?

**Answer** _____

Answers on page 182
Score **1 point** for each correct answer   Your score _____

## 19 WHAT TIME IS IT? II

Minutes are counted in base 60. Try using base 60 with the following:

**A** You finished a 10 kilometre run in 1 hour 12 minutes. Your running partner finished 24 minutes ahead of you. You both started at 10:11am. What time did your partner cross the finishing line?

**Answer** _____

**C** The time is 4:48pm. You put the dinner in the oven to cook for 90 minutes, but have to check it at two equal intervals. At what times should you check?

**Answer** _____

**B** You are late for an appointment. The bus you are travelling on is 6 minutes delayed. You were already running 17 minutes late. It will take another 18 minutes to arrive at your destination. It is now 9:36am. What time is your appointment?

**Answer** _____

**D** The film *Hours and Minutes* starts at 7:13pm in the Village Cinema. The same film is showing at 7:37pm at the City Cinema. Not including the 7 minute walk to the train station, it takes 12 minutes to get to the City and 21 minutes to get to the Village. The time is now 6:41pm. Which cinema can you arrive at first?

**Answer** _____

Answers on page 182
Score **1 point** for each correct answer   Your score _____

## 20 MISSING NUMBER

Can you work out the missing number?

| 3 | 8 | 11 |
| 5 | 4 | 9 |
| 6 | 7 | 13 |
| 2 | ? | 11 |

MISSING

**Answer** _____

Answer on page 182
Score 1 point for a correct answer
Your score _____

## 21 CURRENCY CONVERTER

You're visiting four countries in four weeks, and you need to change currency for each country. Using the exchange rates below, can you work out all the conversions, without using a calculator?

**1 US$ = GB£0.5**
**1 GB£ = 1.25 Euros**
**1.25 Euro = 100 Yen**
**1 Yen = US$0.02**

**A** What is £400 in $? _____

**B** What is 250 Euros in £? _____

**C** What is 1250 Yen in £? _____

**D** What is $400 in Euros? _____

**E** What is £250 in Yen? _____

**Answers on page 182**

Score 2 points for each correct answer
Your score _____

## 22 WEIGHTS AND MEASURES

The metric system is quite easy to use when it comes to mental arithmetic, but the imperial system can be tougher. Using a calculator, can you convert from one to the other?

Remember:
**1 kilogram = 2.2 pounds**　**1 inch = 2.54 centimetres**
**1 metre = 1.0936 yards**　**1 ounce = 28.35 grams**
**1 foot = 30.5 centimetres**　**1 stone = 14 pounds**

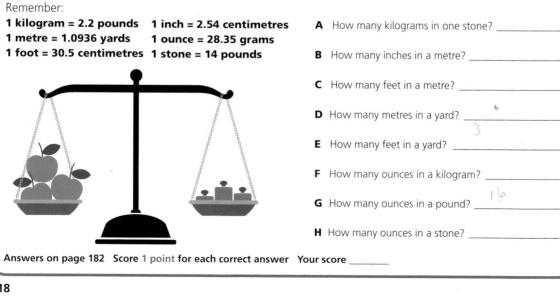

**A** How many kilograms in one stone? _____

**B** How many inches in a metre? _____

**C** How many feet in a metre? _____

**D** How many metres in a yard? _____

**E** How many feet in a yard? _____

**F** How many ounces in a kilogram? _____

**G** How many ounces in a pound? _____

**H** How many ounces in a stone? _____

Answers on page 182　Score 1 point for each correct answer　Your score _____

## 23 BARGAIN BIKE HUNTER

You are looking for a new bike, and you find the same model on offer at two shops, but at a different price in each one. You offer each shop £200 for the bike. The first shop says they'll split the difference and let you have the bike for halfway between your offer and the original price. The second shop says they'll take off 20% from the original price and deduct another £10 on top. If the total of the two original asking prices was £750 and the total of the two final offers is £570, which shop is offering the best price?

**Answer** _____

Answer on page 182
Score 1 point for the correct answer   Your score _____

## 24 DJ BATTLE

You asked Wilfred and Miles to DJ at your party, but you have only one album with 15 tracks on it. Wilfred wants to run a playlist that starts at track 4 and skips two tracks at a time. Miles wants to start his playlist near the end of the album and then work backwards playing every fourth track. Both playlists are four tracks long. If the total of the track numbers in Miles' playlist is six fewer than Wilfred's total, which track is in both playlists?

**Answer** _____

Answer on page 182
Score 1 point for the correct answer   Your score _____

Your score   /70

**60–70 GOLD**

You are skilled at mental arithmetic. Move on to the next chapter to see if you can meet the challenge of more advanced numerical reasoning puzzles.

**30–59 SILVER**

You are fairly numerate, but perhaps you struggled with some of the tougher questions. Have another go at them, using a paper and pen and a calculator if necessary. Learning how to work out the correct answer is often most of the challenge with such problems – once you've cracked that, finding the answer is just a matter of mental arithmetic.

**0–29 BRONZE**

Numerical reasoning can be challenging, but don't let the mere sight of numbers put you in a spin. Try out the Challenge and practise mental arithmetic, then come back and try these exercises again.

★ Turn to page 179 for the Challenge.

## CHAPTER 9

# THE FEAR OF ALL SUMS

## ADVANCED NUMERACY

# The fear of all sums

Although mathematics anxiety is a common problem, the puzzles in this chapter can be solved with the same reasoning and reflection as those in other chapters. Build up your confidence as you tackle them and you can overcome maths anxiety.

## QUESTIONNAIRE
Take this quick quiz to test your mathematical morale.

**1** Imagine that you want to take a course at evening class. One of the courses is in a topic that interests you, but it includes some statistics. Would you still choose it or look for something else?

**Choose it/No thanks**
[score **1 point** for **"Choose it"**]

**2** A friend is struggling to balance her accounts and asks you to take a look at her accounts book. Would you be likely to agree or demur?

**Agree/Demur**
[score **1 point** for **"Agree"**]

**3** On a team-building exercise you are tasked with working out the height of a tree using a long piece of string and a calculator. Would you have a go or rely on another team member rising to the challenge?

**Have a go/Ask someone else**
[score **1 point** for **"Have a go"**]

**4** Your 12-year-old nephew asks for help with his maths homework. Would you be willing to have a look or throw up your hands in horror?

**Look/Horror**
[score **1 point** for **"Look"**]

**5** A society of which you are a member asks you to consider filling the post of treasurer. Would you be likely to give it a try or run a mile?

**Try/Run**
[score **1 point** for **"Try"**]

**6** An estate agent comes round to value your house. She asks you to work out the area of the property in square metres. Would you be likely to succeed or fail?

**Succeed/Fail**
[score **1 point** for **"Succeed"**]

**How did you score?**
**0–2:** It seems you have a bad case of maths anxiety. Have a go at this chapter – the first few exercises at least. The more you exercise your numerical reasoning the more confidence you will have to tackle tougher questions.

**3–4:** You are frightened of maths. Put your faculties to the test with the exercises in this chapter.
**5–6:** Maths holds no terrors for you. Test your mettle with the exercises in this chapter and see if you can do the toughest ones.

# 1 CALCULATOR CRISIS

The operators (+, −, x, and ÷) on your calculator are missing but you don't have time to buy a new one, so you decide to figure out which of the missing keys corresponds to which operator. You label the gaps A, B, C, and D and try out some calculations, with the following results:

4 **(A)** 3 gives the same as 6 **(B)** 6
2 **(C)** 2 is 4
2 **(D)** 2 is also 4
5 **(C)** 7 is less than 8 **(D)** 2
Which button is which?

A _____
B _____
C _____
D _____

**Answers on page 182**
**Score 1 point if you got all the buttons correct**
Your score _____

# 2 PRIME TIME

Prime numbers are numbers that cannot be divided by any other number except 1 and themselves: 1, 3, 5, 7, 11, and so on. Can you work out the next 10 prime numbers after 11?

**Prime numbers** _____

**Answers on page 182**
**Score 3 points if you got them all correct**
Your score _____

# 3 SHARED SECRET

With your prime numbers to hand, what do the following numbers have in common?

25
35
51
77
119
143

**Answer**_____

**Answer on page 182**

**Score 1 point for a correct answer**
Your score _____

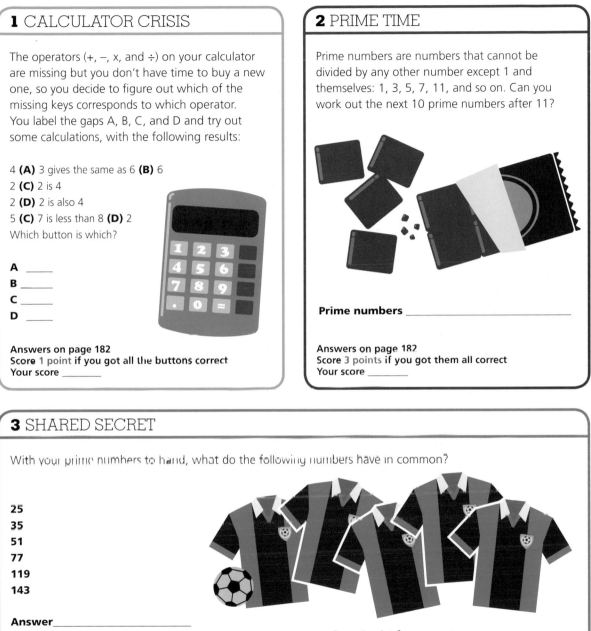

TIP

Try your hand at number-based puzzles in newspapers and magazines. Strictly speaking, puzzles such as Sudoku and Kakuro involve logical rather than numerical reasoning (although they feature numbers, they could equally feature any form of symbols), but there are other puzzle types you can find that exercise your numeracy, such as number puzzles, "side-by-side", and "secret number".

## **4** AVERAGE APPLES

You are working at a greengrocer and you take delivery of a crate of apples. You want to work out the average weight of an apple in the crate, but you have only the information shown on the label in the right. Can you work out the average weight of an apple in the crate?

Answer _____

Answer on page 182
Score **2 points** for a correct answer
Your score _____

Crate contains:
67 apples weighing 112g each
32 apples weighing 98g each
125 apples weighing 132g each
16 apples weighing 102g each

## **5** NUMBER TRIANGLE I

Can you work out a formula, using the three outer numbers of the first triangle below, that gives you the number in the middle of the triangle? Once you have established the formula, use it to work out the missing number in the third triangle.

8
70
7         14

9
74
7         11

7
65
7         ?

Answer_____

Answer on page 182

Score **1 point** for a correct answer   Your score _____

## **6** NUMBER TRIANGLE II

What is the missing number?

Answer on page 182

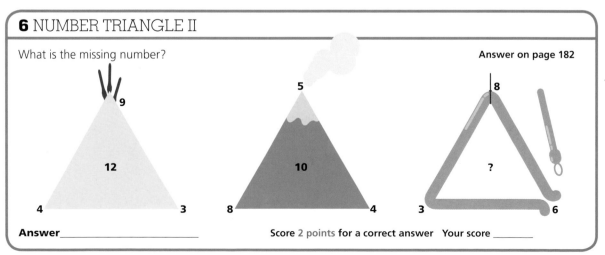

9
12
4         3

5
10
8         4

8
?
3         6

Answer_____

Score **2 points** for a correct answer   Your score _____

## **7** NUMBER CROSS I

What is the missing number?

Answer on page 183

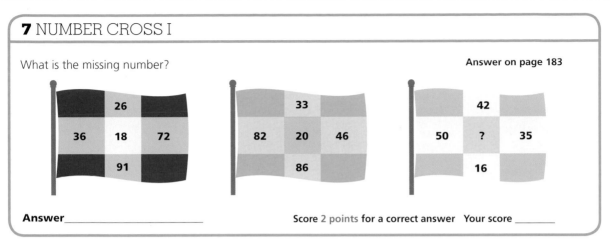

**Answer**_____

Score 2 points for a correct answer   Your score _____

## **8** NUMBER CROSS II

What is the missing number?

Answer on page 183

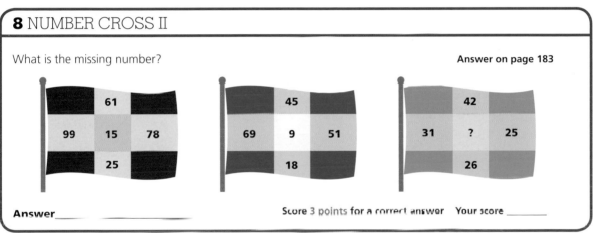

**Answer**_____

Score 3 points for a correct answer   Your score _____

## **9** NUMBER PENTAGON

What are the missing numbers?

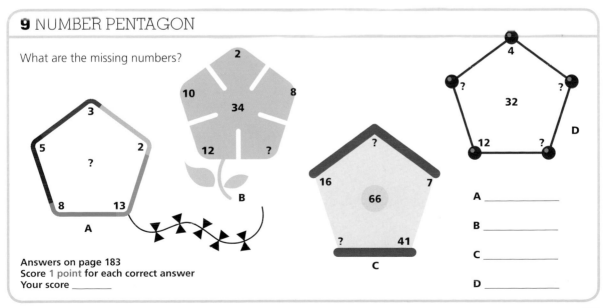

A _____

B _____

C _____

D _____

Answers on page 183
Score 1 point for each correct answer
Your score _____

## **10** NUMBER SQUARE

What is the missing number?

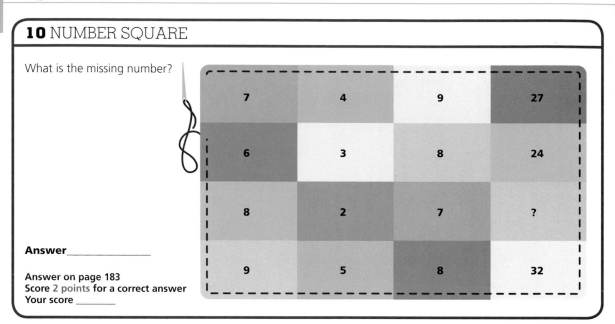

Answer_____

Answer on page 183
Score **2 points** for a correct answer
Your score _____

## **11** WHERE ANGLES FEAR TO TREAD

One of the basic principles of geometry is that the angles of a triangle add up to 180°. You may also recognize right-angle triangles – triangles in which one angle is 90°. Armed with this information, can you work out the missing angles in these triangles? Note these angles are not drawn to scale.

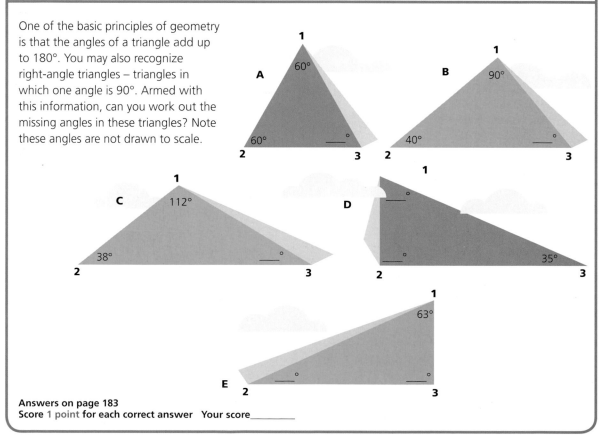

Answers on page 183
Score **1 point** for each correct answer   Your score_____

## 12 IN THE AREA

Here are some formulae for areas of two-dimensional shapes. Can you use them to work out the areas and volumes of the shapes given? For the purposes of this exercise, pi has a value of 3.14.

**Area of a rectangle**
= width x height

**Area of a triangle**
= ½ x base x height

**Area of a circle**
= pi x radius²

**Circumference of a circle**
= 2 x pi x radius

**A**

What is the area of this rectangle? _____

**B**

What is the area of this triangle? _____

**C**

This rectangle has an area of 20. What is its height?

_____

**D**

This triangle has an area of 8. What is its height?

_____

**E**

What is the area and circumference of this circle?

_____

**F**

What is the area and circumference of this circle?

_____

Answers on page 183
Score **1 point** for each correct answer   Your score _____

## 13 FLOOR SPACE

It's your first day on the job as an estate agent and you are sent to measure up a bungalow. Can you use the floorplan below to work out the total area of the house? Each square is 0.5m².

**Answer** _____

Answer on page 183
Score **2 points** for a correct answer   Your score _____

## 14 ALGEBRA ALERT

Algebra is simpler than it looks and, without realizing, you are probably using it on a daily basis. Can you work out what the letter "a" equals in these simple equations?

**A** You've bought 7 apples for a total cost of £3.50. How much does each apple cost? **a x 7 = 350** _____

**B** Your designer tells you that three rolls of fabric will be enough to cover nine armchairs with 2 square metres of fabric each. How many square metres is each roll?
**3a ÷ 9 = 2** _____

**C** Mrs Thruppet donates four boxes of cat food to the pet charity drive, and Mrs Roundel donates three boxes of cat food. The pet charity ends up with 21 tins of cat food. How many tins were in each box? **4a + 3a = 21** _____

**D** Five equally crewed fishing boats left harbour last night, and although all the fishermen make it back alive, only three boats limped back into port the next morning, along with 10 bedraggled fishermen swimming behind them. How many fishermen crew each boat? **5a = 10 + 3a**
_____

**E** Three packets of gum contain as many sticks of gum as 48 divided by the number of sticks of gum in a packet. How many sticks of gum are in a packet? **3a = 48 ÷ a**
_____

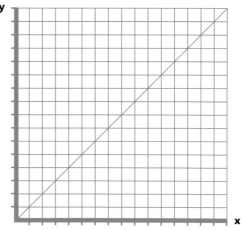

**Answers on page 183**
**Score 1 point for each correct answer**
**Your score _____**

## 15 PLOT IT

Algebra comes in handy for describing lines on graphs. You can also turn real life scenarios into graphs: any situation in which one variable changes according to another one, and numbers are involved, can be plotted. For instance, the algebraic equation x = y shows that every time one unit is added along the x axis, one unit is also added along the y axis (see graph below). Using a separate piece of graph paper, can you plot the lines that correspond to the simple equations that arise from these scenarios.

**Line 1:** You are cycling up a steep hill, gaining 1 metre of altitude for every 2 metres you travel. Draw a graph representing the slope of the hill. **x = 2y**

**Line 2:** Your uneconomical car does 2 miles to the gallon. Plotting the distance (in miles) on the y axis and gallons of fuel on the x axis, graph out your cumulative fuel consumption with the distance as **2x = y**

**Line 3:** Your brother is two years older than you. Draw a graph of his age on the y axis against yours on the x axis. **y = x + 2**

**Answers on page 183**
**Score 1 point for each correct graph.**
**Your score _____**

# 16 LEARNING CURVE

Simple algebraic equations can also be used to represent curved lines on graphs. For example, you could plot a graph of the width of a square carpet on the x axis against its area on the y axis: $y = x^2$. Every time the width, which is the x coordinate, increases by a unit, the area will increase by that unit squared and this will be the y coordinate. The graph below shows the curved line representing the equation $y = x^2$.

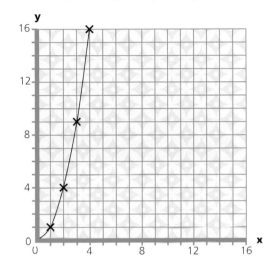

On a separate piece of graph paper, can you now draw a graph with the area of a square room plotted on the x axis and the width of the room on the y axis $y = x^2 - 2$.

**Answer on page 183**
**Score 2 points for drawing the curve correctly**

Your score _____

**TIP**

If you feel that topics such as algebra and geometry are alien, you might want to consider revisiting some basics. There are many websites you can visit that offer easy and engaging ways to reacquaint yourself with maths, from the basics through to more advanced mathematics, helping you build your confidence so you can tackle serious sums without fear.

Your score          /50          **40–50 GOLD**          **20–39 SILVER**          **0–19 BRONZE**

Your mathematical skills are good but did you get 50 out of 50? If you didn't get some of the answers, can you work out where you went wrong?

You had a good crack at the questions but perhaps your maths skills could do with a brush up. Revisit the questions you got wrong.

Possibly your confidence is low, and perhaps you didn't try some of the exercises, or maybe you gave up on them too easily? Keep trying these puzzles until you can answer all of them.

★ Turn to page 179 for the Challenge.

CHAPTER 10
# TIP OF THE TONGUE
## VERBAL INTELLIGENCE

# Tip of the tongue

Verbal acuity, or verbal intelligence, is the ability to use and understand words and language. Your ability results from a combination of your knowledge of language, such as your breadth of vocabulary, and your capability in applying it.

## QUESTIONNAIRE
Use this quick quiz to get an overview of your verbal abilities.

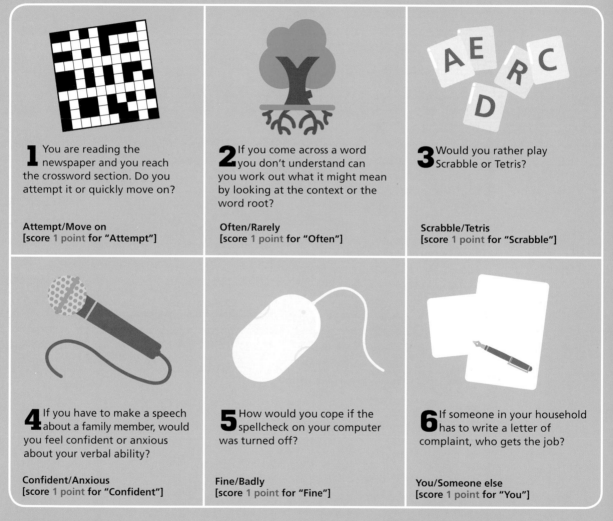

**1** You are reading the newspaper and you reach the crossword section. Do you attempt it or quickly move on?

Attempt/Move on
[score 1 point for "Attempt"]

**2** If you come across a word you don't understand can you work out what it might mean by looking at the context or the word root?

Often/Rarely
[score 1 point for "Often"]

**3** Would you rather play Scrabble or Tetris?

Scrabble/Tetris
[score 1 point for "Scrabble"]

**4** If you have to make a speech about a family member, would you feel confident or anxious about your verbal ability?

Confident/Anxious
[score 1 point for "Confident"]

**5** How would you cope if the spellcheck on your computer was turned off?

Fine/Badly
[score 1 point for "Fine"]

**6** If someone in your household has to write a letter of complaint, who gets the job?

You/Someone else
[score 1 point for "You"]

**How did you score?**

**0–2:** You have little or no confidence in your verbal acuity. Work through the exercises in this chapter to examine your verbal intelligence and give your verbal skills a thorough workout.

**3–4:** Your verbal intelligence is not bad, but there are areas you need to work on. Go through the exercises to find the areas you need to strengthen.

**5–6:** You are articulate and literate, but verbal intelligence and knowledge can always be improved – use the exercises in this chapter to test yourself and hone your abilities.

## 1 FROM A TO Z ⏱

Allow yourself 30 seconds to arrange these 10 words in alphabetical order. Write the appropriate number, from 1 to 10, next to each word.

mouse ___

bottle ___

ladder ___

xylophone ___

zip ___

apple ___

crown ___

wristwatch ___    headphones ___    tree ___

**Answer on page 183**
**Score 1 point for the correct order**
**Your score** _____

## 2 FROM S TO S ⏱

Here is a much tougher alphabetizing challenge. Allow yourself 30 seconds to arrange these 10 words into alphabetical order. Write the appropriate number, from 1 to 10, next to each word.

___ **seduction**          ___ **sedan**

___ **sedation**           ___ **sedentary**

___ **sedimentation**      ___ **sedimentary**

___ **sedulous**           ___ **sedative**

___ **seditious**          ___ **seductive**

**Answer on page 183**
**Score 3 points for the correct order**
**Your score** _____

## 3 FILL IN THE GAPS

Below is a story told in pictures. Can you place the words supplied on the right into the blank spaces so that they make sense and tell a story?

**ignored; until; guarded; shook; squawking; but; arrived**

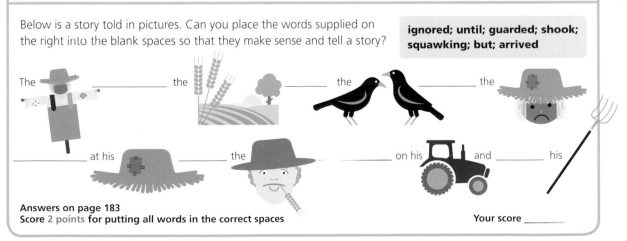

The ___ _____ the ___ _____ the ___ _____ the ___

_____ at his ___ _____ the ___ _____ on his ___ and _____ his

**Answers on page 183**
**Score 2 points for putting all words in the correct spaces**

**Your score** _____

133

## 4 SYNONYMS

Synonyms are words with the same or similar meaning. In the four lists of words below, circle the two that are the most similar in meaning.

**A**

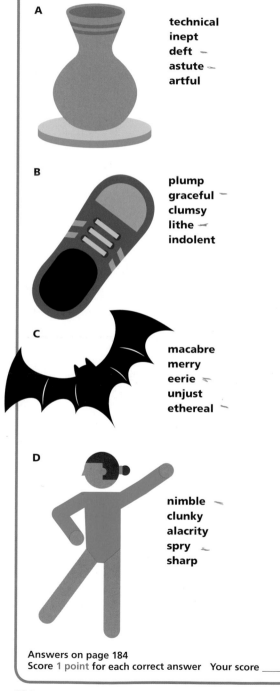

technical
inept
deft
astute
artful

**B**

plump
graceful
clumsy
lithe
indolent

**C**

macabre
merry
eerie
unjust
ethereal

**D**

nimble
clunky
alacrity
spry
sharp

Answers on page 184
Score **1 point** for each correct answer   Your score _____

## 5 SYNONYMS BY ANALOGY

In each of the following, circle the correct analogy that would make the statement true.

**A**

**loneliness** is to **isolation** as **deception** is to:
malice
mendacity
ingeniousness
errancy

**B**

**robust** is to **sturdy** as **flimsy** is to:
heavy
feckless
fanciful
fragile

**C**

**flag** is to **pennant** as **signal** is to:
waving
semaphore
alarmed
ignore

**D**

**alert** is to **ready** as **honest** is to:
exhibition
vigilant
virtuous
circus

Answers on page 184
Score **1 point** for each correct answer   Your score _____

# 6 ANTONYMS

An antonym is a word that is opposite in meaning to another. In each of the lists below, circle the two words that are the most opposite in meaning.

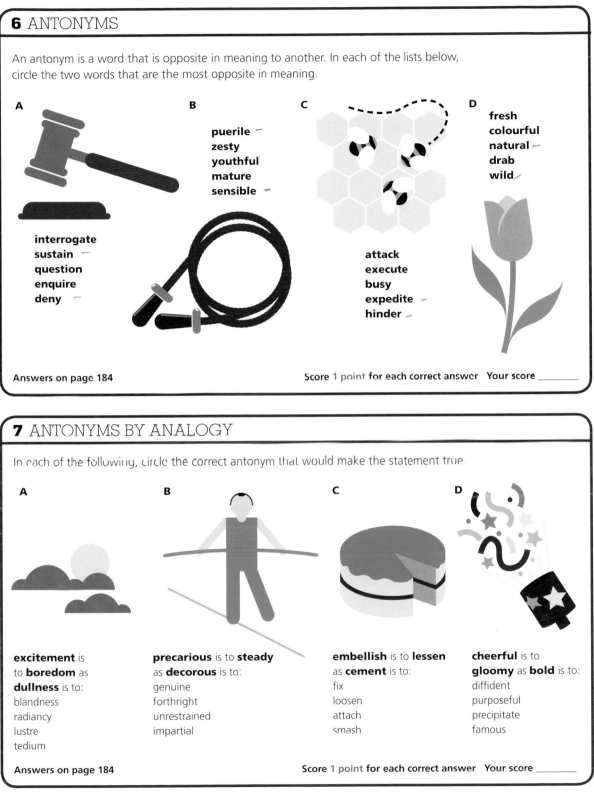

**A**

interrogate
sustain —
question
enquire
deny —

**B**

puerile —
zesty
youthful
mature
sensible —

**C**

attack
execute
busy
expedite —
hinder —

**D**

fresh
colourful
natural —
drab
wild —

Answers on page 184

Score 1 point for each correct answer   Your score _____

# 7 ANTONYMS BY ANALOGY

In each of the following, circle the correct antonym that would make the statement true.

**A**

**excitement** is to **boredom** as **dullness** is to:
blandness
radiancy
lustre
tedium

**B**

**precarious** is to **steady** as **decorous** is to:
genuine
forthright
unrestrained
impartial

**C**

**embellish** is to **lessen** as **cement** is to:
fix
loosen
attach
smash

**D**

**cheerful** is to **gloomy** as **bold** is to:
diffident
purposeful
precipitate
famous

Answers on page 184

Score 1 point for each correct answer   Your score _____

## 8 LETTER COUNTING

Here are 20 letters with their values. Using any number/combination of these letters, can you make words with these exact scores?

**A  16** _____

**B  23** _____

**C  17** _____

**D  8** _____

Answers on page 184

**Score 2 points for each score you managed**  Your score _____

## 9 WORD GRID

Find the hidden 12-letter word by finding the starting letter and moving between adjacent letters in a horizontal or vertical direction only – no diagonal moves allowed. Use each letter only once. You need to guess any missing letters.

| | | | |
|---|---|---|---|
| E | R | T | |
| V | P | | V |
| E | | T | E |

**Answer** _____

Answer on page 184
**Score 1 point for a correct answer**  Your score _____

## 10 ODD ONE OUT

**A** Which group of letters is the odd one out?

**INGTRAIN**
**ILEMOB**
**FULSIN**
**PLAINFAST**
**MEALWHOLE**

**Answer** _____

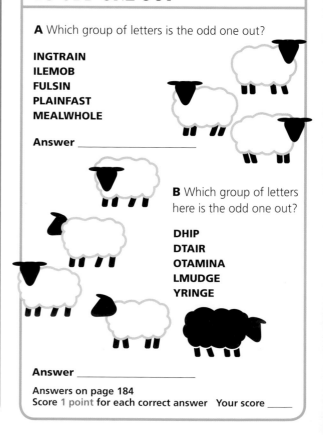

**B** Which group of letters here is the odd one out?

**DHIP**
**DTAIR**
**OTAMINA**
**LMUDGE**
**YRINGE**

**Answer** _____

Answers on page 184
**Score 1 point for each correct answer**  Your score _____

## 11 STROOP TEST

The Stroop Test is a fun verbal assessment of how your perception and verbal intelligence work together, showing how unconscious processing can interfere with and even override your conscious intentions. On the right is a box of paint colours, but the words themselves are in a different colour. Try saying aloud, as fast as you can, the colour of each word, not what the word actually says. The part of your brain that processes the meaning of a word still works without your conscious intention, even when you are trying to think and say something else – in this case, what colour the word is written in.

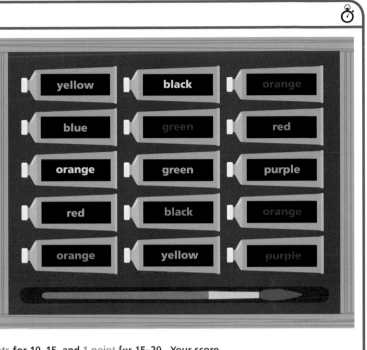

| yellow | black | orange |
| blue | green | red |
| orange | green | purple |
| red | black | orange |
| orange | yellow | purple |

**Score 3 points for less than 10 seconds, 2 points for 10–15, and 1 point for 15–20   Your score** _____

## 12 UPSIDE-DOWN READING

Reading upside down text is a good way to stretch your ability to recognize letters and words, and makes a useful exercise for sharpening your verbal acuity. Without turning it round, quickly scan the passage on the right once and then cover it and answer the questions below.

The Musée du Louvre has a history extending back to medieval times. First constructed as a fortress in 1190 by King Philippe-Auguste to protect Paris against Viking raids, it lost its imposing keep in the reign of François I, who replaced it with a Renaissance-style building. Thereafter, four centuries of kings and emperors improved and enlarged it. A glass pyramid designed by I M Pei was added in 1989.

**A** What was the Louvre's original purpose?   _____

**B** Which king changed the building to Renaissance-style?   _____

**C** Who designed the glass pyramid?   _____

**Answers on page 184**

**Score 1 point for each correct answer   Your score** _____

## 13 WORD LADDERS

Get from the word on the bottom rung to the word on the top rung by changing one letter at a time to form a new (real) word for each rung of the ladder. For instance, you could get from GLUM to FREE by going GLUM > GLUE > FLUE> FLEE > FREE. Time yourself how long it takes to get from the bottom of the ladder to the top.

A    LIE      B    FINE      C    WANE      D    SHEEP

RAY      MAUL      SLIP      BLAND

Score **2 points** for completing each ladder in under 20 seconds, **1 point** for completing in under 30 seconds.
Your score _____

## 14 WORDS WITHIN WORDS

How many words of three or more letters can you make in 5 minutes by using letters from each of the long words below?

**professional**

**creationism**

**illustrated**

**admittance**

**peregrination**

**rhetorical**

**Total number of words** _____

Score **3 points** for 80 plus words, **2 points** for 50–79 words, and **1 point** for up to 50 words in total
Your score _____

**TIP**

A good way to continually increase the breadth of your vocabulary is to make a point of learning at least one new word every day. Whenever you come across a new word, look it up and then make sure you use it in a sentence as often as you can to help fix it firmly in your memory.

## 15 FRUIT SALAD

Which one of these is not an anagram of a fruit? Unscramble all the anagrams to discover which is the odd one out.

**A**  ANA BAN

**B**  FARE PIG RUT

**C**  A CRUEL WOLF I

**D**  EARN MET OWL

**E**  TRACK CAN BLUR

**F**  PLAIN PEEP

**G**  ELECT MEN IN

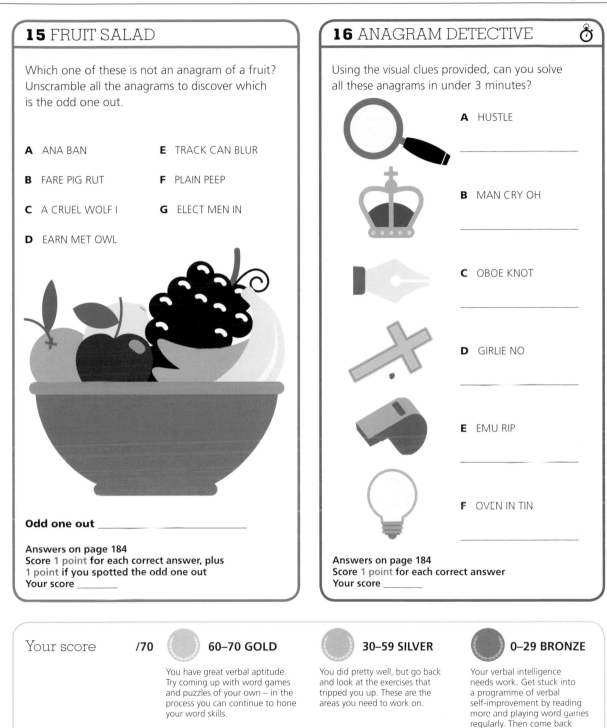

**Odd one out** _____

Answers on page 184
Score **1 point** for each correct answer, plus
**1 point** if you spotted the odd one out
Your score _____

## 16 ANAGRAM DETECTIVE ⏱

Using the visual clues provided, can you solve all these anagrams in under 3 minutes?

**A**  HUSTLE
_____

**B**  MAN CRY OH
_____

**C**  OBOE KNOT
_____

**D**  GIRLIE NO
_____

**E**  EMU RIP
_____

**F**  OVEN IN TIN
_____

Answers on page 184
Score **1 point** for each correct answer
Your score _____

---

Your score   **/70**   ● **60–70 GOLD**

You have great verbal aptitude. Try coming up with word games and puzzles of your own – in the process you can continue to hone your word skills.

● **30–59 SILVER**

You did pretty well, but go back and look at the exercises that tripped you up. These are the areas you need to work on.

● **0–29 BRONZE**

Your verbal intelligence needs work. Get stuck into a programme of verbal self-improvement by reading more and playing word games regularly. Then come back and work through these exercises again.

★ Turn to page 179 for the Challenge.

## CHAPTER 11

# LOST IN SPACE

VISUO-SPATIAL INTELLIGENCE

# Lost in space

Visuo-spatial intelligence or aptitude is the form of intelligence you use when thinking about physical shapes, distances, angles, and sizes in the real world. You use this for example when packing tins into a cupboard or when playing games such as Tetris.

## QUESTIONNAIRE
Do this quick quiz to see how visuo-spatially aware you are.

**1** Would you be able to fit differently shaped items into a small cupboard, or would you just hope they don't fall out when you next open the cupboard door?

**Fit/Fall out**
[score **1 point** for "Fit"]

**2** If you were driving your car and you came to a narrow passage not much wider than your vehicle, would you risk it or find a different route?

**Risk/Avoid**
[score **1 point** for "Risk"]

**3** When using a map to find your way, do you have to turn the map round to line up with the streets or can you do the rotation in your head?

**Turn map round/Rotate in head**
[score **1 point** for "Rotate in head"]

**4** You're ordering a new carpet, but the salesman needs to know the approximate floor area of your living room. Would you try to estimate it or would you need to get out the tape measure?

**Estimate/Measure**
[score **1 point** for "Estimate"]

**5** You're out hiking with a friend and he unfolds the map to check your location, then hands it back to you for folding. Will the map end up perfectly pressed or folded roughly?

**Pressed/Roughly**
[score **1 point** for "Pressed"]

**6** The sun is out and you set up the deckchair. Can you snap it into shape without difficulty, or will you have to wrestle with it like an angry anaconda?

**Snap/Wrestle**
[score **1 point** for "Snap"]

### How did you score?
**0–2:** Sounds as though you're struggling a little with your visuo-spatial intelligence. Work through all the exercises to help improve your ability.

**3–4:** Your visuo-spatial intelligence is average, but you sometimes lack confidence. Use the exercises in this chapter to put your visuo-spatial acuity through its paces and prove that you can do it.

**5–6:** You have an acute sense of visuo-spatial awareness. Put your capacity to the test and see if you can complete all the challenges in the chapter without too much pondering.

# 1 SPOT THE DIFFERENCE

Below are two apparently identical pictures. In fact, there are six differences between the two – can you spot them all? Time how long it takes you.

**Answer on page 184**

Less than 1 minute: score 3 points, less than 2 minutes: 2 points, more than 2 minutes: 1 point **Your score** _____

# 2 FLOOR PLANNER

You have a new job as a carpet fitter. If each side of the squares on the floorplan below is 0.5m, can you work out how many square metres of carpet in total you will need for the rooms? The hall and the stairs are to remain uncarpeted.

**Answer** _____

**Answer on page 184**

Score 2 points for a correct answer **Your score** _____

## 3 GET YOUR HEAD AROUND THIS

Mental rotation (the ability to turn an image in your mind's eye accurately enough so that you can correctly perceive its elements relative to one another) is a key marker of visuo-spatial aptitude, and a popular puzzle in IQ tests. Here is a relatively simple example to get you started. These squares are identical but rotated, with one exception. Which is the odd one out?

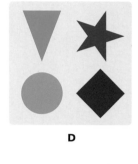

| **A** | **B** | **C** | **D** |

**Answer** _____    Answer on page 184    Score **1 point** for a correct answer   Your score _____

## 4 AMBASSADORIAL AMBUSH

Now challenge your mental rotation ability further. As the new ambassador for Ruritania, you are hosting your first diplomatic function, but the etiquette department have placed the flags the wrong way round, and slipped in one from a different country for good measure. Below is what the Ruritanian flag looks like the right way round. Which of the flags on the right is the not the Ruritanian flag?

**A**            **B**

**C**            **D**

**Answer** _____    Answer on page 184    Score **1 point** if you identified the correct flag   Your score _____

## 5 TOUGH ROTATION

Here is a more taxing mental rotation test. Which of the pentagons below is the odd one out?

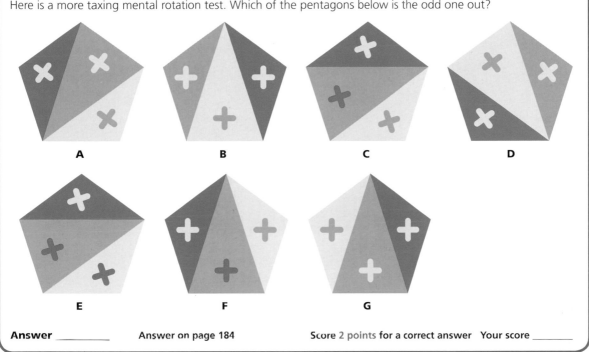

| A | B | C | D |

| E | F | G |

Answer _____     Answer on page 184          Score 2 points for a correct answer   Your score _____

## 6 ABOUT FACE

Below are three views of the same cube. Use your mental rotation ability to work out which side is opposite pattern D?

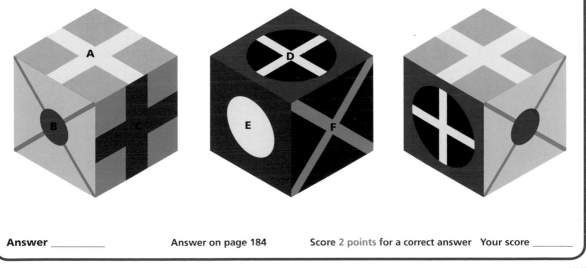

Answer _____          Answer on page 184          Score 2 points for a correct answer   Your score _____

145

## 7 A CUBE WITH A VIEW

Which of the cubes below is not a view of the same cube?

**A**

**B**

**C**

**D**

**E**

**Answer** _____

## 8 UNPACKING

If you "unfold" the sides of a cube, laying them flat to make a two-dimensional shape, you get a cross shape such as the one shown below.

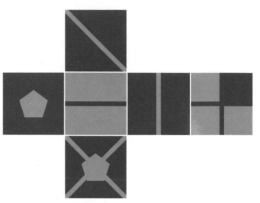

Which of the following is the cube that you can make by folding up this cross?

**A**

**B**

**C**

**D**

**E**

**Answer** _____

Answer on page 185
Score 2 points for the correct answer

Your score _____

## **10** MAP MAKER

Using this list of landmarks and the links between them listed below, can you draw an accurate map?

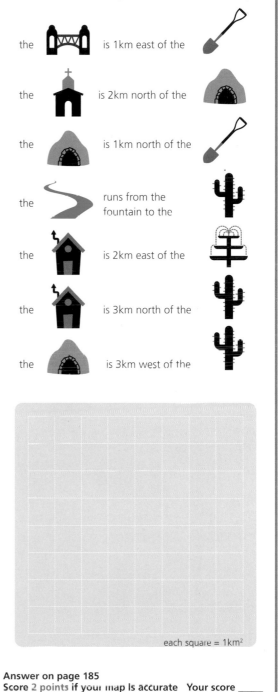

the [bridge] is 1km east of the [shovel]

the [church] is 2km north of the [cave]

the [cave] is 1km north of the [shovel]

the [river] runs from the fountain to the [cactus]

the [hut] is 2km east of the [fountain]

the [hut] is 3km north of the [cactus]

the [cave] is 3km west of the [cactus]

each square = 1km²

> **TIP**
>
> Three-dimensional mental rotation can be quite a challenge. One way to cope is to break down the problem into more manageable aspects. For instance, when dealing with a cube, pick a face and label it in your mind as "Top", then note the relationship between the top face and the ones on either side of it. Do the same with other views, so that all you are trying to visualize at any one time is the relationship between three elements.

## **9** WHERE IN THE WORLD?

You are hiking in the mountains. The picture below shows the view you can see. Based on the features and topography visible, can you locate yourself on the map beneath it?

**Answer on page 185**
**Score 2 points** if you located yourself correctly
**Your score** _____

**Answer on page 185**
**Score 2 points** if your map is accurate   **Your score** _____

## 11 FREEZER PACKER

A load of shopping has just been delivered, and you have the unenviable task of cramming it into the chest freezer. Can you work out the best configuration and sketch the shapes of the packets below onto the diagram of the freezer?

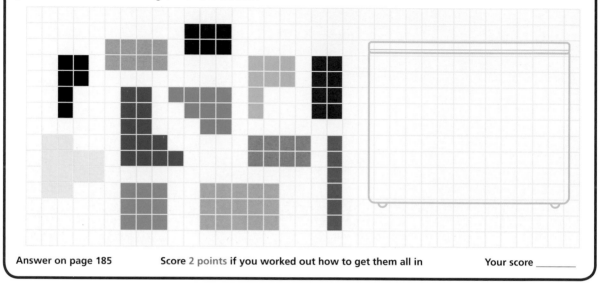

Answer on page 185          Score 2 points **if you worked out how to get them all in**          Your score _____

## 12 TILE GAME

You have a tile game where any adjacent tile can be moved up or down into the empty space. It currently looks like this:

Which of the following can't you make?

A          B          C

D          E          **Answer** _____

Answer on page 185
**Score 1 point for a correct answer  Your score _____**

## 13 CHESS MOVES

The key on the left shows a knight chess piece can move to any of the squares indicated with a black dot. On the board below, what is the least number of moves needed for the knight to take the stationary rook?

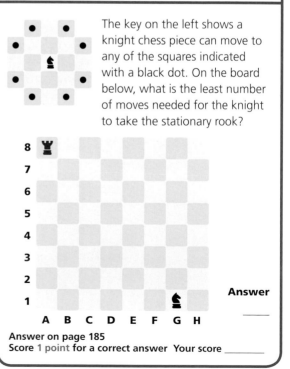

**Answer**
_____

Answer on page 185
**Score 1 point for a correct answer  Your score _____**

# 14 SHAPES SERIES I

Look at the following sequence of four and decide which of the three options below comes next in the series.

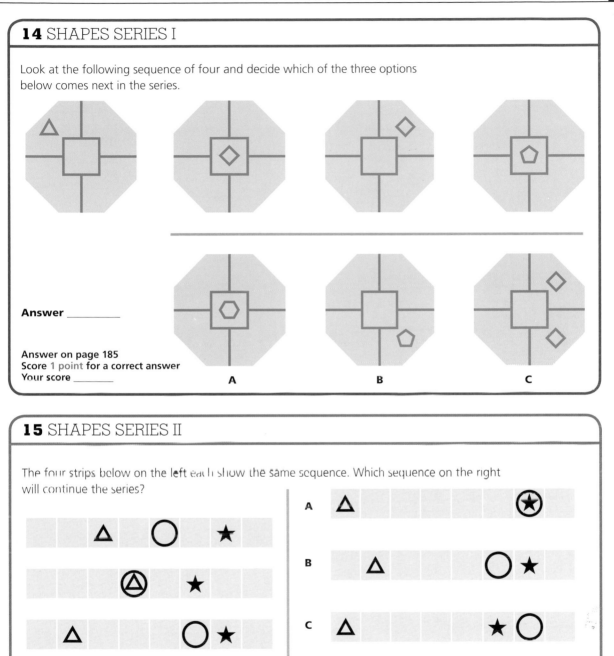

**Answer** _____

Answer on page 185
Score 1 point for a correct answer
Your score _____

A          B          C

# 15 SHAPES SERIES II

The four strips below on the left each show the same sequence. Which sequence on the right will continue the series?

**Answer** _____

Answer on page 185
Score 1 point for a correct answer  Your score _____

## **16** STRIKE A POSE

Look at the sequence of movements.

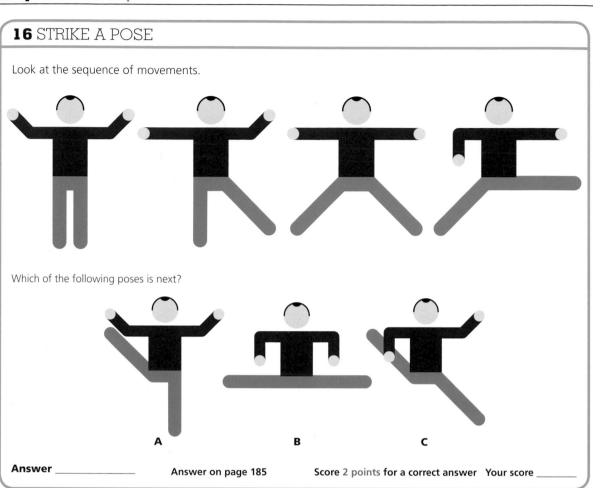

Which of the following poses is next?

A          B          C

**Answer** _____          **Answer on page 185**          **Score 2 points for a correct answer   Your score** _____

## **17** TELLTALE SHAPES I

Look at the series of shapes below. The colours tell you something about the shapes.

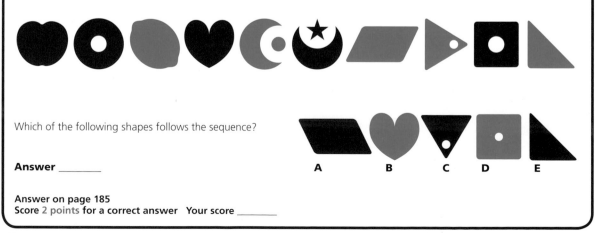

Which of the following shapes follows the sequence?

**Answer** _____

A          B          C          D          E

**Answer on page 185**
**Score 2 points for a correct answer   Your score** _____

## 18 TELLTALE SHAPES II

Look at the sequence on the right.

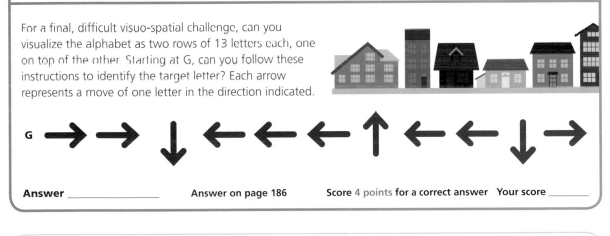

Which of the following comes next in the series?

**A**

**B**

**C**

**D**

**Answer** _____

**Answer on page 185**

**Score 2 points** for a correct answer   **Your score** _____

## 19 ALPHABET STREET

For a final, difficult visuo-spatial challenge, can you visualize the alphabet as two rows of 13 letters each, one on top of the other. Starting at G, can you follow these instructions to identify the target letter? Each arrow represents a move of one letter in the direction indicated.

G → → ↓ ← ← ← ↑ ← ← ↓ →

**Answer** _____

**Answer on page 186**

**Score 4 points** for a correct answer   **Your score** _____

Your score   **/40**

**30–40 GOLD**

Your performance on these exercises is impressive. Take a look at the ones where you stumbled and work on those aspects of visuo-spatial intelligence.

**20–29 SILVER**

Some of the tougher exercises caused you problems. Go back and work through them again. Familiarize yourself with this sort of puzzle to try to improve your performance.

**0–19 BRONZE**

Mental rotation puts your head in a spin. Check out the Challenge to see how you can work on your visuo-spatial aptitude in everyday life.

Turn to page 179 for the Challenge

# Logic jam

Logical intelligence involves your powers of reasoning – thinking through problems in a methodical, step-by-step way. However, the human brain is not wired for this kind of thinking, so most people use intuition and mental shortcuts in reasoning. A key to success in logic tests is to think about the exact wording of the question.

## QUESTIONNAIRE

Can you avoid logical fallacies and see through codes and cyphers, or do you tend to stumble into logical pitfalls and struggle to break codes? Use this quick quiz to find out how logical your brain is.

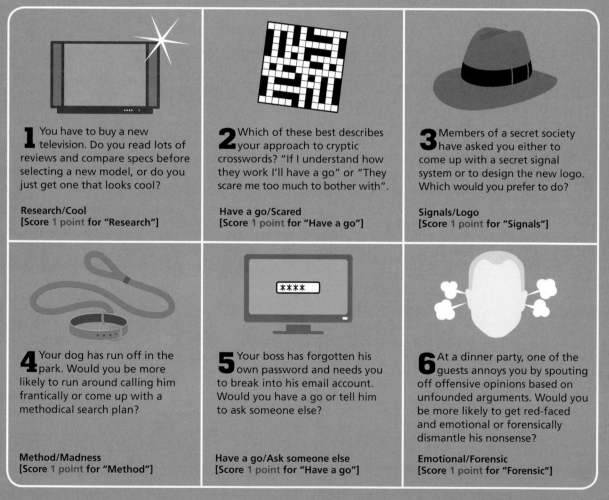

**1** You have to buy a new television. Do you read lots of reviews and compare specs before selecting a new model, or do you just get one that looks cool?

**Research/Cool**
[Score 1 point for "Research"]

**2** Which of these best describes your approach to cryptic crosswords? "If I understand how they work I'll have a go" or "They scare me too much to bother with".

**Have a go/Scared**
[Score 1 point for "Have a go"]

**3** Members of a secret society have asked you either to come up with a secret signal system or to design the new logo. Which would you prefer to do?

**Signals/Logo**
[Score 1 point for "Signals"]

**4** Your dog has run off in the park. Would you be more likely to run around calling him frantically or come up with a methodical search plan?

**Method/Madness**
[Score 1 point for "Method"]

**5** Your boss has forgotten his own password and needs you to break into his email account. Would you have a go or tell him to ask someone else?

**Have a go/Ask someone else**
[Score 1 point for "Have a go"]

**6** At a dinner party, one of the guests annoys you by spouting off offensive opinions based on unfounded arguments. Would you be more likely to get red-faced and emotional or forensically dismantle his nonsense?

**Emotional/Forensic**
[Score 1 point for "Forensic"]

### How did you score?

**0–2:** You tend to think with your heart not your head, but do not despair. Many logical-thinking techniques can be learned easily and are down to practice. If you struggle, try to learn from your mistakes.

**3–4:** You try to approach problems logically, but sometimes you fall into the trap of irrational thinking. Try to bear in mind that gut instinct can lead you astray.
**5–6:** You are as logical as Spock, but can you master all the challenges in this chapter?

## 1 WHICH ANIMAL IS NEXT?

The four animals below follow a sequence.

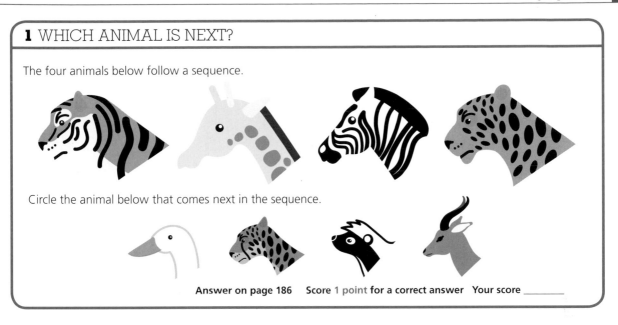

Circle the animal below that comes next in the sequence.

Answer on page 186    Score 1 point for a correct answer   Your score _____

## 2 MATERIAL WORLD

Which of the options listed on the right is the most logical one to continue this sequence?

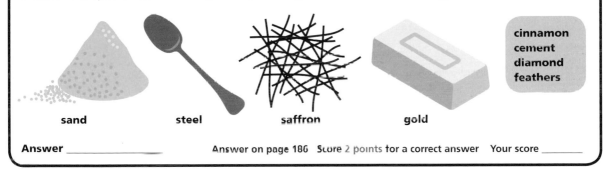

sand        steel        saffron        gold

cinnamon
cement
diamond
feathers

Answer _____    Answer on page 186   Score 2 points for a correct answer   Your score _____

## 3 THE DAY TODAY

The day before the day before yesterday is three days after Saturday. What day is it today?

Answer _____

Answer on page 186   Score 1 point for a correct answer   Your score _____

## **4** ALPHABET DIRECTIONS

Look at the letters below. Circle the letter that is to the right of the letter third to the left of the letter that (in the alphabet) comes after the letter that, below, is second to the left of T?

R   H   V   Y   S   A   I   T   B   N

**Answer** _____     Answer on page 186   Score 1 point for a correct answer   Your score _____

## **5** REASONING BY ANALOGY

Select the number below that best completes the analogy **9** is to **6** as **12** is to…?

**A** 6

**B** 10

**C** -12

**D** 8

**E** 4

**Answer** _____     Answer on page 186   Score 1 point for a correct answer   Your score _____

## **6** PEACE MAKER

**165135** is to **peace** as **129225** is to:

**A** plenty

**B** love

**C** live

**D** abacus

**Answer** _____

Answer on page 186
Score 1 point for a correct answer   Your score _____

## **7** COFFEE TIME

**Coffee** is to **5566153** as **apple** is to:

**A** 193572

**B** 51216161

**C** 216169

**D** 1937722

**Answer** _____

Answer on page 186
Score 1 point for a correct answer   Your score _____

## 8 LAW AND ORDER

Arrange the words below in a logical sequence.

**arrest**

**parole**

**prison**

**crime**

**court**

**thief**

Answer _____

_____

Answer on page 186
Score 1 point for a correct answer   Your score _____

## 9 ANIMAL PLANET

Arrange the words below in a logical order.

**mammal**

**beaver**

**herbivore**

**animal**

**vertebrate**

**rodent**

Answer _____

_____   _____

Answer on page 186
Score 1 point for a correct answer   Your score _____

## 10 AIR AND SEA

Arrange the words below in a logical order.

**dinghy**

**kite**

**submarine**

**jet**

**airship**

**hydrofoil**

Answer _____

Answer on page 186   Score 1 point for a correct answer   Your score _____

## 11 MUSICIANS' UNION

These Venn diagrams represent an orchestra. The circle labelled C represents players of string instruments. The circle labelled U represents musicians who are members of a union. The head of the union plays a tuba. In which of the diagrams does the shaded area include him?

**Answer** _____    **Answer on page 186   Score 1 point for a correct answer   Your score** _____

## 12 SPORTS CLUB

All the kids at sports club play at least one of the three sports on offer: football, tennis, or volleyball. On the Venn diagram, shade in the areas that show children who either play one sport only, or those who play all three.

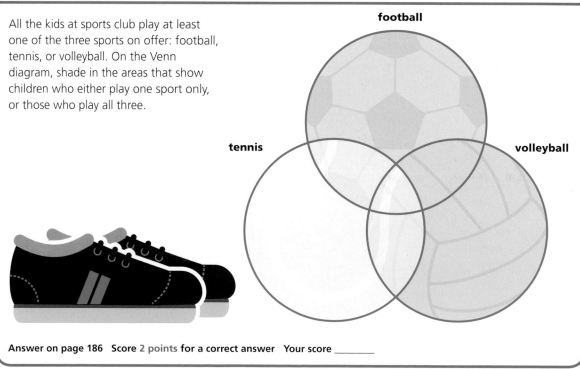

**Answer on page 186   Score 2 points for a correct answer   Your score** _____

## 13 INTERVIEW CHOICE

There are 20 people who have applied for a job. Of these, 15 are women and 8 are shortlisted. Everyone who applied is either a woman or has been shortlisted. How many women were shortlisted? Drawing a Venn diagram on a separate piece of paper can help you work out the answer.

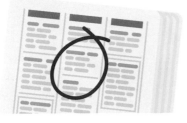

**Answer** _____

Answer on page 186
Score 2 points **for a correct answer  Your score** _____

## 14 DAMAGED GOODS

At an auction you buy a job lot of 20 vinyl records, which are a mixture of albums and singles, but 6 of them are scratched. Of the records, 8 are albums. If there are 8 singles that are not scratched, how many of the albums are scratched? Drawing a Venn diagram on a separate piece of paper can help you work out the answer.

**Answer** _____

Answer on page 186
Score 2 points **for a correct answer  Your score** _____

## 15 PIRATE SHIP

Out of 32 suspects captured from a pirate's ship:

5 pirates were arrested for wearing an eyepatch, having a wooden leg, and carrying a parrot on their shoulders.

3 pirates were arrested for wearing an eyepatch, having a wooden leg, but didn't carry a parrot on their shoulders.

9 pirates were not arrested for wearing an eyepatch, did not have a wooden leg, and didn't carry a parrot on their shoulders.

11 pirates were arrested for wearing an eyepatch and carried a parrot on their shoulders.

16 pirates were arrested for wearing an eyepatch.

9 pirates with wooden legs carried a parrot on their shoulders.

13 pirates had a wooden leg.

**How many pirates carried a parrot on their shoulder?**
Draw a Venn diagram on a separate piece of paper to work out the answer.

**Answer** _____     Answer on page 186   Score 3 points **for a correct answer  Your score** _____

## 16 TRUE OR FALSE? I

Either Suzy has a driving licence or Suzy isn't allowed to drive. Suzy doesn't have a licence, so she isn't allowed to drive.

**True or false?**

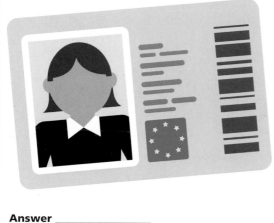

Answer _____

Answer on page 186
Score 1 point for a correct answer  Your score _____

## 17 TRUE OR FALSE? II

If I am shorter than Bill, then Bill is tall. Bill is tall. Therefore I am shorter than Bill.

**True or false?**

Answer _____

Answer on page 186
Score 1 point for a correct answer  Your score _____

## 18 TRUE OR FALSE? III

At the school concert some of the students are playing in the orchestra. The students who are in the orchestra are musically gifted. Some of the students will go on to study at the Conservatory. Students who win a place at the Conservatory are musically gifted. Based solely on these statements, students who are playing in the orchestra will go on to study at the Conservatory.

**True or false?**

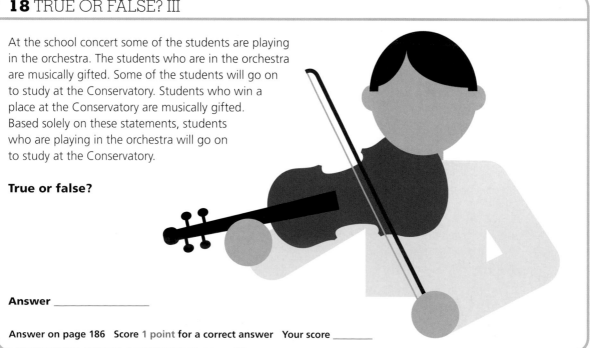

Answer _____

Answer on page 186   Score 1 point for a correct answer   Your score _____

## 19 WHICH IS NEXT?

**SPARKLE**     **LANGUISH**     **STUDENT**     **NEPOTISM**     **SECURE**

Which of the following words should come next?

**IRRADIATE**

**REGULAR**

**MEDICAL**

**FINISHED**

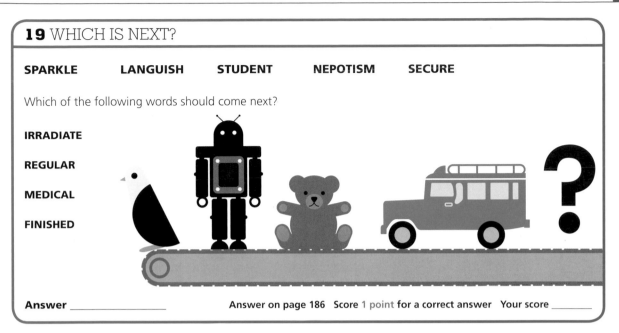

Answer _____     Answer on page 186   Score 1 point for a correct answer   Your score _____

## 20 LETTER LOGIC I

Circle the group of letters that is the odd one out.

**BCDFGH**

**STUWXY**

**EFGIJK**

**DEFIJK**

**MNOQRS**

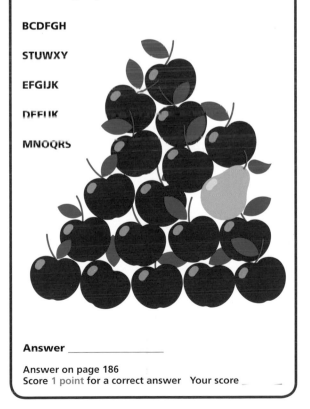

Answer _____

Answer on page 186
Score 1 point for a correct answer   Your score _____

## 21 LETTER LOGIC II

Circle the group of letters that is the odd one out.

**QRTYP**

**FGHKL**

**QDVHO**

**ZVBNM**

**ASDJL**

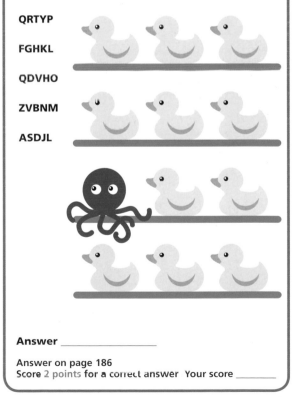

Answer _____

Answer on page 186
Score 2 points for a correct answer   Your score _____

## 22 MEDAL CONFUSION

Your friends Tanya and Brendan have just come back from a sports event and are telling you about who won the medals in the 800m final, but they seem a little confused. Tanya says that Owembe got the gold and Beaker got the silver, but Brendan insists that Armitage won the gold and Owembe got the silver. It turns out that while Owembe, Beaker, and Armitage did indeed share the three medals, neither Tanya nor Brendan was completely accurate – each got one of the medals right and one wrong. Who actually won each of the medals?

**Gold** _____

**Silver** _____

**Bronze** _____

**Answer on page 186   Score 2 points for a correct answer   Your score _____**

## 23 WHICH CARD?

Look at the four cards below. You are not allowed to turn over more than two of them. Which should you turn over to find out whether the following hypothesis is true: "Of the cards shown, any card with a vowel on one side has an even number on the other side."

E          6          9          F

**Answer** _____

**Answer on page 186   Score 2 points for a correct answer   Your score _____**

## 24 SOCK SELECTOR

You have 20 pairs of socks: 10 pairs of purple socks and 10 pairs of red socks. However, they are not paired up, meaning there are 40 loose socks in your sock drawer. With your eyes closed, how many socks do you need to pull out of the drawer to ensure that you end up with at least one matched pair?

**Answer** _____

Answer on page 186
**Score 1 point** for a correct answer   Your score _____

## 25 FESTIVE FOUL-UP

You've bought three boxes of chocolates as presents for your grandmother, uncle, and niece: a box of toffee centres for your niece, who is allergic to alcohol; a box of chocolate liqueurs for granny, who doesn't like toffee; and a mixed box for your uncle who likes both. Disaster strikes, however, as the sweet shop has put the wrong labels on all three boxes. You don't want to ruin the packaging more than necessary, but neither do you want to give the wrong box to the wrong person. Which box or boxes should you open so that you can try a chocolate, in order to make sure everyone gets the right present?

**Answer** _____

Answer on page 187
**Score 2 points** for a correct answer   Your score _____

## 26 LETTER CHANGER

Letter substitution can be used when code writing (see Caesar Cypher, below), but can also be used for a simple word puzzle. In the example below, for the words on either side of the blank space the same letter can be used to replace the second letter of each word to give two new words. Write this letter in the space provided; together the replacement letters spell out a famous name.

| ACES | _____ | AJAR |
|------|-------|------|
| BIDE | _____ | BUCK |
| ORYX | _____ | ACTS |
| EMIT | _____ | ISLE |
| SPUN | _____ | CLIP |
| PACK | _____ | LUCK |

Answers on page 187   Score 1 point for each correct answer   Your score _____

## 27 CAESAR CYPHER

Decryption of codes is a specific application of logical aptitude. One of the simplest forms of code writing is letter substitution, where one letter is replaced with another. The simple cypher supposedly employed by Julius Caesar is created by simply shifting one or more letters to the right in the alphabet, so that, in a single-shift cypher for instance, A is written as B, B as C, and so on. In a triple-shift cypher, A→D, B→E, and so on. Given the specified shifts, decode the cypher texts below and reveal their true meaning.

| | Shift | Cypher text | Answer |
|---|-------|-------------|--------|
| A | 1 | SPNBOT | _____ |
| B | 2 | YJKURGT | _____ |
| C | 2 | JKFFGP | _____ |
| D | 3 | VHFUHW | _____ |

Answers on page 187
Score 1 point for each decryption   Your score _____

## 28 SECRET MESSAGE

Can you use a triple-shift Caesar cypher to encode this message?

**URGENT MESSAGE, MEET CONTACT TONIGHT**

**Answer**_____

Answer on page 187
Score 2 points for encoding correctly  Your score ___

## 29 BLACK AND WHITE

Below are the names of five black-and-white animals, encoded using a Caesar cypher. Can you work out the shift of the cypher from the cypher text, and identify all the animals?

**RCPFC** _____

**BGDTC** _____

**UMWPM** _____

**DCFIGT** _____

**RGPIWKP** _____

**Shift** _____

Answers on page 187
Score 1 point for identifying each animal and 1 point for working out the shift  Your score _____

## 30 SPOT THE E

Here is a cypher text written in a Caesar cypher. Can you use frequency analysis of the letters (see Tip, below) to decipher the following cypher?

**JQJAJS JQJUMFSYX JCNYJI YMJ JQJAFYTW JCHQFNRNSL JCHNYJIQD**

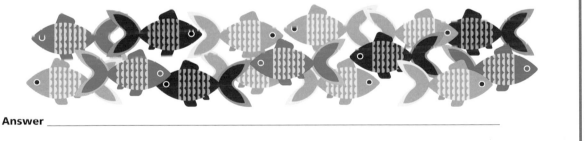

**Answer** _____

Answer on page 187   Score 2 points for a correct answer  Your score _____

TIP

When trying to break a code, there are things you can look out for. For example, in most languages some letters are much more common than others: in English the most common letter is E; 12.7% of letters in a typical English text are the letter E. The next most common letter in English is T, with a frequency of 9.1%. Breaking a code by counting the letters is known as "frequency analysis".

## 31 MORSE CODE

Morse code was invented to allow transmission of letters and numbers by simple pulses of sound/electricity. Using the chart on the right, can you translate the following words into Morse code?

A  MIND _____

B  TRAIN _____

C  SPEAR _____

D  BUFFALO _____

| A | B | C | D | E | F | G |
|---|---|---|---|---|---|---|
| .- | -... | -.-. | -.. | . | ..-. | --. |

| H | I | J | K | L | M | N |
|---|---|---|---|---|---|---|
| .... | .. | .--- | -.- | .-.. | -- | -. |

| O | P | Q | R | S | T | U |
|---|---|---|---|---|---|---|
| --- | .--. | --.- | .-. | ... | - | ..- |

| V | W | X | Y | Z | | |
|---|---|---|---|---|---|---|
| ...- | .-- | -..- | -.-- | --.. | | |

Answers on page 187   Score **1 point** for **4/4**   Your score _____

## 32 EMERGENCY TRANSMISSION

You are operating the wireless on a ship sailing across the Pacific when you pick up this message. Using the chart in exercise 31, can you decode it? (Forward slashes indicate the break between words.)

... --- ... / ... .... .. .--. .-- .-. . -.-. -.- . .-.. / --- -. / -.-. --- .-. .- .-.. / .. ... .-.. . -. -. ..

Answer _____

Answer on page 187   Score **2 points** for a correct answer   Your score _____

## 33 RIVER BOAT CROSSING

You have to transport a fox, a chicken, and a bag of corn across a river. On each trip across the river your boat can only carry you and one of the others, but the problem is that if you leave the fox with the chicken, or the chicken with the corn, one of them will get eaten. How do you get all three to the other side of the river?

**Answer** _____

_____

_____

Answer on page 187

**Score 3 points for a correct answer   Your score** _____

## 34 INTO THE DESERT

You need to deliver a message from Fort Beau to Fort Geste, which takes six days of travel across arid, scorching desert. You have three camels and two other legionnaires to help you, but each camel can only carry enough water to last itself and a rider for four days. What is the minimum number of camels you need to deliver the message safely to Fort Geste without leaving yourself or any other legionnaires stranded in the desert?

**Answer** _ _____

_____

_____

Answer on page 187

**Score 3 points for a correct answer  Your score** _____

Your score     **/70**     **60–70 GOLD**

You are able to approach problems logically, focusing clearly on what the questions are asking and thinking through your answers. See the Challenge for ways to be logical in daily life.

**30–59 SILVER**

You are succeeding up to a point, but possibly the harder questions are tripping you up. Try the Challenge for tips on how to practise logical thinking.

**0–29 BRONZE**

Your logic reasoning needs work. Possibly you rushed to give your answers without properly thinking them through, or let yourself be overwhelmed by the problems. Try them again using methodical reasoning.

Turn to page 179 for the Challenge.

CHAPTER 13
# SPARK OF GENIUS
CREATIVITY

# Spark of genius

Pinning down the definition and mechanism of creativity is difficult, but research has shown ways in which creativity can be stimulated and lubricated. This chapter introduces a variety of exercises designed to stimulate and/or unblock the creative powers you already possess, as well as looking at how to boost them further.

## QUESTIONNAIRE

Is your mind alive with vistas of visionary splendour or do you daydream about spreadsheets? Answer the questions in this quick quiz to find out just how creative you are.

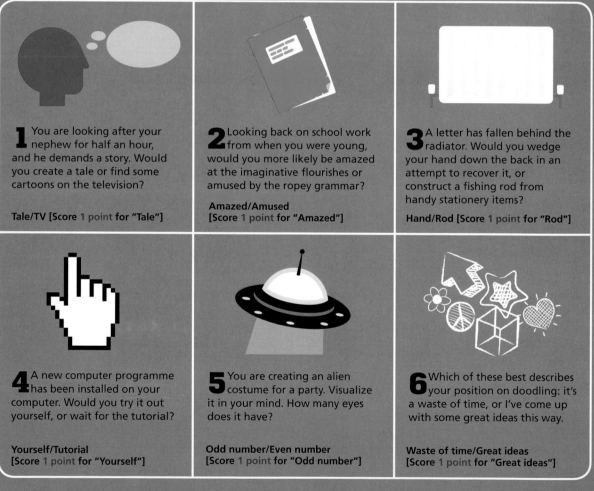

**1** You are looking after your nephew for half an hour, and he demands a story. Would you create a tale or find some cartoons on the television?

**Tale/TV [Score 1 point for "Tale"]**

**2** Looking back on school work from when you were young, would you more likely be amazed at the imaginative flourishes or amused by the ropey grammar?

**Amazed/Amused
[Score 1 point for "Amazed"]**

**3** A letter has fallen behind the radiator. Would you wedge your hand down the back in an attempt to recover it, or construct a fishing rod from handy stationery items?

**Hand/Rod [Score 1 point for "Rod"]**

**4** A new computer programme has been installed on your computer. Would you try it out yourself, or wait for the tutorial?

**Yourself/Tutorial
[Score 1 point for "Yourself"]**

**5** You are creating an alien costume for a party. Visualize it in your mind. How many eyes does it have?

**Odd number/Even number
[Score 1 point for "Odd number"]**

**6** Which of these best describes your position on doodling: it's a waste of time, or I've come up with some great ideas this way.

**Waste of time/Great ideas
[Score 1 point for "Great ideas"]**

**How did you score?**
**0–2:** You think of yourself as a straightforward type. This doesn't mean you don't have creative potential, simply that you are not used to unleashing it. The exercises in this chapter could help.

**3–4:** You have innate creativity, but you are probably not aware of the simple tricks you can use to boost this. Work through the exercises in this chapter to find out more.
**5–6:** You have a powerful imagination. See how original you can be as you work through this chapter.

# 1 ONE WORD FITS ALL

The ability to use the same word in different contexts or, better still, in constructions of widely divergent meaning, is a marker of creativity, and particularly of creative faculty with language. It is known as the "remote associates" test. Psychologists use this exercise to test a person's creativity. For each of the word triplets below, can you find a word that fits with all of them to make a recognized phrase or word? For example, if you had the words "sleep", "way", and "moon", the answer would be "walk".

citrus

bowl

fly

mark

shelf

worm

wall

lime

clip

news

party

march

word

engine

fire

**Answers on page 187**

# 2 CREATIVE CATEGORIZATION

Creativity is sometimes characterized as the ability to make new connections, especially connections that are not obvious or familiar. Try out this aspect of creativity by coming up with new ways to connect the objects shown below by organizing them into groups in novel and unexpected ways. How many ways of categorizing them can you come up with in 5 minutes? Try to make the categories as original as possible.

## 3 THINK OF THE OPPOSITE

A popular creativity-stimulating exercise that forces you to think in novel ways and challenge preconceptions is to conceptualize opposites. This exercise can be used for everything from marketing strategies to technological goals. Stimulate your grey matter by coming up with an opposite to the following concepts. There are no right or wrong answers, but don't mistake "absence of" for "opposite" – for instance, the opposite of gravity is not "weightlessness".

**omelette** _____

**design** _____

**diary** _____

**wine** _____

**eagle** _____

## 4 FLIP IT

Related to finding the opposite is turning on its head your "normal thinking" about something. This forces you into novel conceptualizations. On a separate piece of paper, write down the five reasons requested in each scenario below.

You inherit a sum of money from a relative. Give five reasons why this is bad news.

You are at a restaurant and your main course is delicious and served at just the right temperature. List five reasons why you would send it back.

Getting out of the shower you slip and break your ankle. Give five reasons why you are lucky this happened.

You have a pile of dirty laundry to do. List five reasons why this is good news.

## 5 ALTERNATIVE USES

The standard test in experiments researching factors that influence creativity is called the "alternative uses" test. Your task is to come up with as many alternative uses as possible for an everyday object in a limited time. Try to be as original and imaginative as you can. Allowing 2 minutes for each, see how many alternative uses you can write down on a separate piece of paper for each of these objects:

**paperclip**     **whisk**     **newspaper**     **pencil sharpener**

## 6 DOODLE DESIGN

Doodling is a good way to be creative in an accessible everyday context. It's not the quality of your drawing that counts but the novelty of your design. Explore your creativity here by creating a scene on the grid, right. You must follow these two rules: you can only draw horizontal and vertical lines (no diagonals allowed), and your scene must include all the coloured boxes.

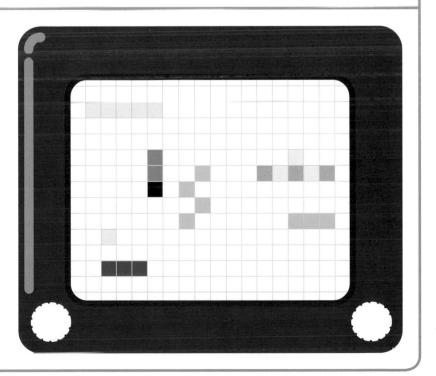

## 7 FANTASTIC VOYAGE

Challenge your creative flair further. A mad inventor has sent you the start of his drawing for a revolutionary new vehicle (see below). Complete the blueprint and design the strangest and most original craft ever to drive, fly, float, or dive – or do all four!

## 8 UNDER THE SEA

Visualize a creature in the murky depths of the ocean. Now sketch it in the space below. Don't read the text at the bottom of the page until you have finished.

How many eyes, arms, tentacles, and such like does your creature have? Is it symmetrical? Research suggests that when creativity is flowing freely, the creatures that people sketch are less symmetrical and less constrained by the rules of terrestrial anatomy.

# 9 JAILBREAK

You are trapped at the top of a tower, with nothing for company except the array of unusual objects pictured below. On a separate piece of paper, see if you can come up with an escape plan that cunningly employs every one of the objects – the more far-fetched and fantastical the better.

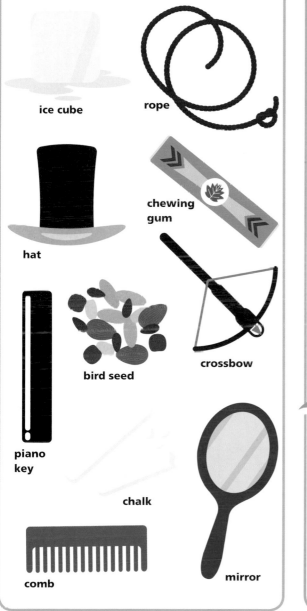

ice cube

rope

hat

chewing gum

piano key

bird seed

crossbow

chalk

comb

mirror

# 10 FAIRY TALE BLITZ

Pressure to create can produce some unusual results. See this for yourself with this exercise. Below are typical elements from a fairy tale. You have 10 minutes to write down, on a separate piece of paper, the plots of three different fairy tales, each involving all of the elements depicted.

princess

frog

apple

tree

spinning wheel

fox

ogre

mirror

bean stalk

## 11 JEOPARDY

Can you work backwards from each of the punchlines below and, on a separate piece of paper, come up with a funny story that leads up to it, using no more than five sentences?

…and that's why you never let a monkey give you a haircut!

…so the sailor says to the king, "I'm sorry, sir, we don't take American Express."

…and the last one to get his shoes back was the Ambassador.

…and the sign said, "You don't have to work here to be mad, but it helps."

## 12 STORY CORNERS

Writers who struggle to get their creative juices flowing sometimes do quick creative writing exercises. Here is an example – the beginning and end of a story are supplied below. On a separate piece of paper, can you write the intervening narrative? You can write as much as you want, but aim for at least 100 words.

It was a dark and steamy night. A shot rang out, and a car slipped quietly out of the warehouse and over the edge of the wharf, into the greasy waters of the Hudson…

…Jerrod put his feet up on the table and took a long drink from a short glass. It had been his toughest case yet, and except for the ruined photographs, the the missing suspect, and the stolen pistol, he thought it had all gone rather well.

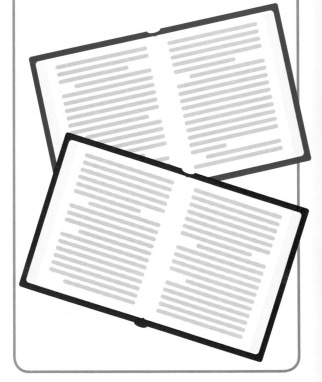

**TIP**

Research shows that the simple technique of putting mental distance between you and a problem can help stimulate creative thinking about the problem. For instance, if you have to solve a problem about someone you work with, think about how another person far away or from a different era might solve the problem. Putting temporal or spatial distance between you and the problem can boost the creativity of your response.

# 13 HOLLYWOOD HOKUM

On a separate piece of paper, come up with titles
and one-line synopses for the following film posters.

## How did you get on?

There is no scoring in this
chapter, so assess yourself
subjectively.

### I WAS INSPIRED

If you found these exercises
inspiring and enjoyable, then
see if you can transfer these skills
to other aspects of intelligence
and use them to enhance your
all-round cognitive performance.
For instance, creative visualization
is a powerful tool for memory-
enhancing performance.

### I DID OKAY

Did some of the exercises inspire
you more than others? Go back
and see what the common
factors were for the tasks that
fired your creativity. Perhaps you
can use these as triggers for
creativity in other scenarios.

### I STRUGGLED

If you found the exercises
difficult and time-consuming,
consider your working
environment when approaching
the tasks. Try out the Challenge
to get into a more creative frame
of mind.

 Turn to page 179
for the Challenge.

# Challenges

How did you find the exercises throughout the book? If your score for a chapter was low, or you felt that you struggled on a certain chapter, then try the relevant Challenge below. Even if you succeeded in the chapters, these Challenges will help to boost your brain power further.

## CHAPTER 1

### INSTANT REVIEW

Practise instant reviewing (immediately going over new information in your head or out loud) so that it becomes a habit. Repeat phone numbers, licence plates, shopping lists, people's names, and such like, on an everyday basis to help to kickstart the transfer of information from STM to intermediate memory, where it won't fade as quickly.

## CHAPTER 2

### THE OTHER HALF

Set yourself the target of memorizing the names of the partners of all the people with whom you share an office or gym class or any suitable group of people you wish. Start off by writing down a list, and then use memory techniques that form associations between the people you know and their partners' names. Test yourself after a week, a month, and three months, and see if you find the names easier to recall after a period of time has passed.

## CHAPTER 3

### DOORSTEP ROUTINE

A good habit to get into is making a house-leaving routine, which you practise on the doorstep before you close the door. Pat your pockets or look inside your bag and run through a mental checklist. Keys? Check! Wallet? Check! Travel pass? Check!

## CHAPTER 4

### BANK REVIEW

A good way to give your MTM a workout is to sit down with an itemized bank statement and work through the cash payments you have made in the last few days or weeks. Cover the place details, leaving only the amounts and the dates and try to recall the relevant locations.

## CHAPTER 5

### DAILY REVIEW

If you're trying to improve your biographical memory, you need to improve your encoding. One tactic is to get into the habit of reviewing your activities and experiences at the end of each day. Without question the best way to do this is to keep a journal, but even if you just take 5 minutes to run through the day's events in your head it should help.

## CHAPTER 6

### NOW YOU SEE IT

Create visualizations for each of your PINs to make them easier to recall. For example, you could link the shape of each number to an object: the number 1 could remind you of a pencil, for example, and the number 4 might make a sailing boat spring to mind. Once you have your objects relating to the numbers, combine them to make one memorable image and practise recalling the image when you need to remember your PIN. You can also incorporate into your visualization the colour of the card the PIN goes with to further boost recollection of which PIN relates to which card.

## CHAPTER 7

### SYSTEM ADDICT

A systematic approach to revision can boost the efficiency and efficacy of learning. Use a 5-stage system. 1. Preview the material by skimming to get an idea of its content. 2. Write a list of questions to answer when you're finished. 3. Read through the material with the goal of finding answers to your questions. 4. Summarize what you've learned by reviewing the main points. 5. Test yourself within 24 hours by writing answers to the questions you posed earlier.

## CHAPTER 8

### CHANGE FOR THE BETTER

Use mental arithmetic whenever paying for something with cash. Get into the habit of mentally totting up the cost of the goods you are buying. Work out in your head the change that will be due when you pay, before the cashier does the calculation for you.

## CHAPTER 9

### PLOT YOUR LIFE

Turn real-world scenarios into graphs. Any situation in which one variable changes according to another, and numbers are involved, can be graphed out. For instance, you could draw a graph of how your salary has changed over time, or how your weight has changed with age. Not only is this good exercise for your numerical intelligence, but it can also give you an interesting new angle on things.

## CHAPTER 10

### LEVEL UP YOUR READING

Improve your vocab and all-round verbal aptitude by reading more books, journals, and newspapers. Keep a notepad and pencil handy and get into the habit of writing down words you don't know and looking up their meanings later. Make a point of trying to use each new word you have learnt in conversation on a regular basis.

## CHAPTER 11

### ANTIPODEAN MOUSE

A simple exercise to get your visuo-spatial processes working (specifically, the activity in the cerebellum, the area at the back of the brain that controls coordination) is to turn your computer mouse through 180° and try creating a picture in a drawing programme with it.

## CHAPTER 12

### LOGIC

Cryptography is a form of logical reasoning – start up an encrypted correspondence with someone, and challenge each other to break codes of your own devising.

## CHAPTER 13

### MEDITATION FOR CREATIVITY

State of mind is believed to be an important influence on creativity and your ability to think creatively. Anxiety and distractions tend to sap creativity, but a clear, focused mind can dramatically enhance it. Set aside 5 minutes every day to sit quietly and observe what is happening around you. Then see if you can create a short story linking events you can see, as your creative thoughts start to surface.

# Answers

## CHAPTER 1

### 2 WHERE DID YOU GET THAT HAT?

The baseball cap is the odd one out as it is the only hat with a peak.

### 6 CAN YOU CUT IT?

### 10 DRAWING WITH YOUR MIND'S EYE

### 11 DUCKS IN A ROW

### 14 TREASURE ISLAND

You end up at the red hut.

### 24 INTERFERING OBJECTS

The escalator is the odd one out as it's the only one that moves you. All the others you have to physically move yourself on.

### 25 INTERFERING NUMBERS

The jack of clubs.

## CHAPTER 3

### 16 LEFT AND RIGHT

You end up at the church.

## CHAPTER 6

### 2 LEETSPEAK

**A** GOBULLDOGS = 9*|3|_|11|)*9$

**B** XYLOPHONE = %'/,1*IO#*|\3

**C** BIRTHDAY = |3!|27#|)@'/,

**D** CALORIES = (@1*|2!3$

**E** WHITEHOUSE = VV#!73#*|_|$3

### 3 STACKED UP

**A** 4046 = rfvp;/rfvyhn

**B** 1979 = qazol.ujmol.

**C** 2005 = wsxp;/p;/tgb

**D** 8238 = ik,wsxedcik,

### 4 BASE SYSTEM

**A** A41A14A

**B** IA16GO17

**C** 3BMSHTR

**D** ATWI80D

## 5 SYSTEM ADDICT
**A** 5TULOB
**B** 7YCAGWYW
**C** 4TKAM
**D** 6RSANSD

## 6 BESPOKE PASSWORDS
**A** gre10TTBBITFOTN
**B** eve10TTBBITFOTN
**C** y3k10TTBBITFOTN
**D** leg10TTBBITFOTN

## 7 CONSONANT SWAP
**A** 10TTEEITFOTN
**B** 10ETEBITUATN
**C** 10TTBBOUFOTN
**D** 10TEBΛITEOTN

## 8 MADE TO MEASURE
**A** gree10TT
**B** even10TT
**C** y3ks10TT
**D** lega10TT

## 11 UP STACKED
**A** 5354
**B** 8902
**C** 6232
**D** 9715

## 15 LETTER PAIRS PLUS
**A** ASPP – 0855
**B** TCJT = 9299
**C** WABO = 2014
**D** EPMG = 4526

## 19 THIS OLD MAN
**A** 2187
**B** 0645
**C** 2934

---

## CHAPTER 7

### 1 QUIZ MASTER
**1** India
**2** Beethoven
**3** Atlantic, Arctic, Indian, Pacific, Southern
**4** "For every action there is an equal and opposite reaction"
**5** China
**6** 1917
**7** Buzz Aldrin
**8** Femur (thighbone)
**9** Uruguay
**10** Walt Disney. He won 26 oscars

### 2 SPOT THE LINK
They are all landlocked countries (they have no coastline)

---

## CHAPTER 8

### 1 ARITHMETIC 101
**A** 1,221
**B** 13,203
**C** 246
**D** 3,274
**E** 693
**F** 6,612
**G** 11
**H** 13

### 2 RAISING CHANGE
**A** £4.15
**B** £1.05
**C** £8.95
**D** £1.02

### 3 PAPERBACK PROBLEM
The Secret Life of Aunts and Year of the Yak (£16.98). Your change will be £0.52.

### 4 CANDY CONUNDRUM
**Answer:** 21

---

## 5 ARE YOU COORDINATED?
**A** X–2, Y–3
**B** X2, Y9
**C** X7, Y5
**D** X4, Y1
**E** X6, Y–4

## 6 GOLDEN BOOTY
There are 600 coins in the wooden chest and 1,400 in the steel chest.

## 7 WHICH IS BIGGER? I
**1** $\frac{7}{8}$
**2** $\frac{3}{4}$
**3** $\frac{2}{3}$
**4** $\frac{9}{16}$
**5** $\frac{2}{5}$
**6** $\frac{5}{15}$

## 8 WHICH IS BIGGER? II
**1** $\frac{9}{12}$
**2** $\frac{2}{3}$
**3** $\frac{5}{8}$
**4** $\frac{6}{10}$
**5** $\frac{9}{15}$
**6** $\frac{15}{32}$

## 9 DECIMALS VS FRACTIONS I
**1** 0.8
**2** $\frac{2}{3}$
**3** 0.6
**4** $\frac{2}{6}$
**5** 0.3
**6** $\frac{1}{4}$

## 10 DECIMALS VS FRACTIONS II
**1** $\frac{11}{21}$
**2** 0.5
**3** $\frac{2}{5}$
**4** 0.333
**5** 0.275
**6** $\frac{7}{32}$

continued ➔

## CHAPTER 8 continued

### 11 SOCK PUZZLE
Answer: 20

### 12 SLICE OF THE PIE
A
1 $\frac{1}{2}$
2 $\frac{1}{4}$
3 $\frac{1}{4}$
B
1 $\frac{1}{4}$
2 $\frac{1}{6}$
3 $\frac{1}{6}$
4 $\frac{1}{6}$
5 $\frac{1}{4}$
C
1 $\frac{1}{3}$
2 $\frac{1}{9}$
3 $\frac{1}{9}$
4 $\frac{1}{9}$
5 $\frac{1}{3}$
D
1 $\frac{1}{4}$
2 $\frac{1}{8}$
3 $\frac{1}{8}$
4 $\frac{1}{4}$
5 $\frac{1}{8}$
6 $\frac{1}{8}$

### 13 STAR STRUCK
Answer: 75% $\frac{3}{4}$ of 160 = 120; 90/120 = $\frac{3}{4}$ (75%)

### 14 LITTLE BROTHER
Answer: 6

### 15 CHEESE PLEASE
A £12.10
B £14.10
C £18.19

### 16 HENRY'S CAT
Answer: 16

### 17 BILL BRAINTEASER
A 10
B 5
C 5
D 5

### 18 WHAT TIME IS IT? I
A 9am
B 1am
C 8pm
D 13 hours; 6pm

### 19 WHAT TIME IS IT? II
A 10.59am
B 10:17am
C 5:18pm and 5:48pm
D City Cinema

### 20 MISSING NUMBER
Answer: 9. The final square in each row is the sum of the first two squares.

### 21 CURRENCY CONVERTER
A $800
B £200
C £12.50
D €250
E 25,000 Yen

### 22 WEIGHTS AND MEASURES
A 14/2.2 = 6.36kg
B 100/2.54 = 39.37in
C 100/30.5 or 39.37/12 = 3.28ft
D 1/1.0936 = 0.9144m
E 3.28 x 0.9144 = 3 ft
F 1,000/28.35 = 35.27oz
G 35.27/2.2 = 16oz
H 16 x 14 = 224oz

### 23 BARGAIN BIKE HUNTER
The second shop. The original price in the first shop is £400, and £350 in the second shop.

### 24 DJ BATTLE
Track 13. Wilfred's playlist is 4, 7, 10, 13, so Miles' must be 13, 9, 5, 1.

## CHAPTER 9

### 1 CALCULATOR CRISIS
A –
B ÷
C +
D x

### 2 PRIME TIME
Answer: 13, 17, 19, 23, 29, 31, 37, 41, 43, 47

### 3 SHARED SECRET
They are all products of prime numbers (5x5 = 25; 3x17 = 51; 7x17 = 119).

### 4 AVERAGE APPLES
Answer: 119.88g. The average is the combined weight of all the apples divided by the total number of apples. The combined weight is found by multiplying the weight categories by the number in each category: (67x112) + (32x98) + (125x132) + (16x102) = 7504+3136+16500+1632 = 28772; total number apples = 240; 28772/240 = 119.88g

### 5 NUMBER TRIANGLE I
Answer: 16. The numbers in the centre are the sum of the bottom right number and the product of the other two numbers: 65 – (7x7) = 16

### 6 NUMBER TRIANGLE II
Answer: 4. The central number is found by dividing the product of the top number and the bottom left number by the bottom right number: (8x3)÷6 = 4

## 7 NUMBER CROSS I

**Answer:** 13. The middle number is the sum of the individual digits of the top and bottom number and also the left and right number: 4+2+1+6 = 13; 5+0+3+5 = 13

## 8 NUMBER CROSS II

**Answer:** 10. The middle number is the difference between the difference between the top and bottom numbers and the difference between the left and right numbers:
(42–26) – (31–25) = 16 – 6 = 10

## 9 NUMBER PENTAGON

In each pentagon, starting from the top right number and top numbers and finishing with the central number, the numbers are the sums of the previous two numbers.
**A** 21 (13+8 = 21)
**B** 22 (34–12 – 22)
**C** 9 and 25 (66–41= 25; 25–16 – 9)
**D** 4, 8, and 20 (32–12 = 20, 20–12 = 8, 8–4 – 4)

## 10 NUMBER SQUARE

**Answer:** 42. In each row, the last column is the product of the third column and the difference between the first two columns:
(8–2) x 7 = 42

## 11 WHERE ANGLES FEAR TO TREAD

**A** 60°
**B** 50°
**C** 30°
**D** 1 = 55°; 2 = 90°
**E** 1 = 27°; 3 = 90°

## 12 IN THE AREA

**A** 24
**B** 9
**C** 4
**D** 4
**E** area = 28.26; circumference = 18.84
**F** area = 50.24; circumference = 25.12

## 13 FLOOR SPACE

**Answer:** 49sqm

## 14 ALGEBRA ALERT

**A** 0.50
**B** 6
**C** 3
**D** 5
**E** 4

## 15: PLOT IT

## 16 LEARNING CURVE

## CHAPTER 10

## 1 FROM A TO Z

**1** apple
**2** bottle
**3** crown
**4** headphones
**5** ladder
**6** mouse
**7** tree
**8** wristwatch
**9** xylophone
**10** zip

## 2 FROM S TO S

**1** sedan
**2** sedation
**3** sedative
**4** sedentary
**5** sedimentary
**6** sedimentation
**7** seditious
**8** seduction
**9** seductive
**10** sedulous

## 3 FILL IN THE GAPS

The scarecrow **guarded** the field **but** the crows **ignored** the scarecrow, **squawking** at his old hat, **until** the farmer **arrived** on his tractor and **shook** his rake.

continued →

## CHAPTER 10 continued

### 4 SYNONYMS
**A** Technical and artful
**B** Graceful and lithe
**C** Eerie and macabre
**D** Nimble and spry

### 5 SYNONYMS BY ANALOGY
**A** Mendacity
**B** Fragile
**C** Semaphore
**D** Virtuous

### 6 ANTONYMS
**A** Sustain and deny
**B** Puerile and mature
**C** Expedite and hinder
**D** Colourful and drab

### 7 ANTONYMS BY ANALOGY
**A** Radiancy
**B** Unrestrained
**C** Loosen
**D** Diffident

### 8 LETTER COUNTING
There are many answers for each amount. Here is an example for each.
**A** TUMBLER
**B** JEOPARDY
**C** EXAMS
**D** HOB

### 9 WORD GRID
PREVENTATIVE

### 10 ODD ONE OUT
**A** PLAINFAST. The others can be made into words by swapping round the syllables.
**B** YRINGE. The others can be made into a word by replacing the first letter with the letter S.

### 12 UPSIDE-DOWN READING
**A** A fortress to protect Paris from Viking attacks.
**B** François I.
**C** I. M. Pei.

### 15 FRUIT SALAD
**A** Banana
**B** Grapefruit
**C** Cauliflower
**D** Watermelon
**E** Blackcurrant
**F** Pineapple
**G** Clementine
Cauliflower (C) is the odd one out as it is the only vegetable.

### 16 ANAGRAM DETECTIVE
**A** Sleuth
**B** Monarchy
**C** Notebook
**D** Religion
**E** Umpire
**F** Invention

## CHAPTER 11

### 1 SPOT THE DIFFERENCE

### 2 FLOOR PLANNER
**Answer:** 47sqm

### 3 GET YOUR HEAD AROUND THIS
**Answer:** D. The others are all rotations. D is a mirror image of C.

### 4 AMBASSADORIAL AMBUSH
**Answer:** B. The red squares have been flipped.

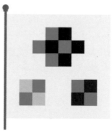

### 5 TOUGH ROTATION
**Answer:** E. The others all have identical pairs in different rotations: A and G; B and D; C and F.

### 6 ABOUT FACE
**Answer:** C

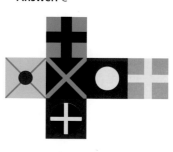

## 7 A CUBE WITH A VIEW
**Answer:** A

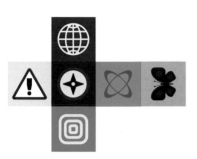

## 8 UNPACKING
**Answer:** D. All the others could be views of the same cube – only in view A does the arrangement of sides not match up with what is shown in the other views.

## 9 WHERE IN THE WORLD?

## 10 MAP MAKER

## 11 FRIDGE PACKER

## 12 TILE GAME
**Answer:** B

## 13 CHESS MOVES
**Answer:** 5

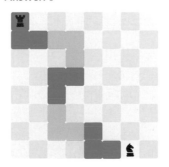

## 14 SHAPE SERIES I
**Answer:** B

## 15 SHAPE SERIES II
**Answer:** A

## 16 STRIKE A POSE
**Answer:** B. The left arm moves down and the right leg moves up by 45°. The right arm then moves down and the left leg up by 45°.

## 17 TELLTALE SHAPES I
**Answer:** C. The purple shapes have a vertical line of symmetry.

## 18 TELLTALE SHAPES II
**Answer:** B. The blue circle is moving along the diagonal, one square at a time; the black circle is shifting left to right; and the triangle is shifting right to left.

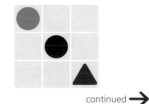

continued →

## CHAPTER 11 continued

### 19 ALPHABET STREET
**Answer:** R

## CHAPTER 12

### 1 WHICH ANIMAL IS NEXT?
Skunk (the sequence is stripes, spots, stripes, spots, so the next animal must be stripy).

### 2 MATERIAL WORLD
Diamond (the sequence goes from least valuable by weight to most valuable).

### 3 THE DAY TODAY
**Answer:** Friday

### 4 ALPHABET DIRECTIONS
**Answer:** I

### 5 REASONING BY ANALOGY
**Answer:** D. 6 is 2/3 of 9, so 2/3 of 12 is 8 (D)

### 6 PEACE MAKER
C: LIVE. The numbers correspond to their position in the alphabet (P=16/26; E=5/26 etc).

### 7 COFFEE TIME
B: 51216161. The numbers correspond to their position in the alphabet, but the answer is backwards (E=5, L=12, P=16, P=16, 1=A).

### 8 LAW AND ORDER
Thief, crime, arrest, court, prison, parole (the logical order of events from first to last).

### 9 ANIMAL PLANET
Beaver, rodent, herbivore, mammal, vertebrate, animal (the classification order).

### 10 AIR AND SEA
Submarine, dinghy, hydrofoil, kite, airship, jet (the order of altitude reached from lowest to highest).

### 11 MUSICIANS' UNION
**Answer:** A

### 12 SPORTS CLUB

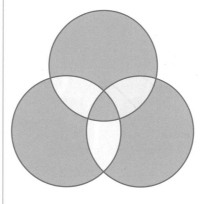

### 13 INTERVIEW CHOICE
**Answer:** 3

### 14 DAMAGED GOODS
**Answer:** 2

### 15 PIRATE SHIP
**Answer:** 17

### 16 TRUE OR FALSE? I
True. This isn't a trick question!

### 17 TRUE OR FALSE? II
False. Bill may be tall, but I may be taller. This fallacy is known as "affirming the consequent": if A, then B is not the same as B, therefore A.

### 18 TRUE OR FALSE? III
False. Just because A therefore C and B therefore C, doesn't mean that A therefore B is correct.

### 19 WHICH IS NEXT?
REGULAR (each word begins with the penultimate letter of the previous word).

### 20 LETTER LOGIC I
DEFIJK. The others skip one letter, this skips two.

### 21 LETTER LOGIC II
QDVHO. The others are all on the same line on a computer keyboard.

### 22 MEDAL CONFUSION
Gold: Armitage; Silver: Beaker; Bronze: Owembe.

### 23 WHICH CARD?
E and 9. Most people try to confirm the hypothesis and choose E and 6. However, the hypothesis doesn't say that an even numbered card must have a vowel on the other side.

### 24 SOCK SELECTOR
**Answer:** 3. If I pull out three socks, at least two of them must be the same colour. Many people mistakenly say 21.

## 25 FESTIVE FOUL-UP

You only need to open the "mixed" box. All the boxes are incorrectly labelled, so the "mixed" box must either be liqueurs or toffee. If it contains liqueurs, you know the box labelled "liqueurs" must contain toffee centres, or else one of the boxes would have the correct label, which we know is not the case.

## 26 LETTER CHANGER

| ACES | [G] | AJAR |
|------|-----|------|
| BIDE | [A] | BUCK |
| ORYX | [N] | ACTS |
| EMIT | [D] | ISLE |
| SPUN | [H] | CLIP |
| PACK | [I] | LUCK |

## 27 CAESAR CYPHER

**A** ROMANS
**B** WHISPER
**C** HIDDEN
**D** SECRET

## 28 SECRET MESSAGE

XUJHQW PHVVDJH PHHW FRQWDFW WRQLJKW

## 29 BLACK AND WHITE

RCPFC [PANDA]
BGDTC [ZEBRA]
UMWPM [SKUNK]
DCFIGT [BADGER]
RGPIWKP [PENGUIN]
This is a double shift cypher.

## 30 SPOT THE E

5 letter shift. The plain text is ELEVEN ELEPHANTS EXITED THE ELEVATOR EXCLAIMING EXCITEDLY.

## 31 MORSE CODE

**A** -- .. -. -..
**B** - .-. .- .. -.
**C** ... .--. . .- .-.
**D** -... ..- ..-. ..-. .- .-.. ---

## 32 EMERGENCY TRANSMISSION

SOS SHIPWRECKED ON CORAL ISLAND

## 33 RIVER BOAT CROSSING

Carry the chicken across first, leave it on the far bank, come back for the corn, drop off the corn and pick up the chicken and take it back to the left bank, swap it for the fox, drop off the fox and come back for the chicken.

## 34 INTO THE DESERT

All three camels set off, but after one day's travel the first camel transfers a day's water to each of the other camels, keeping only the single day's water needed to get back to Fort Beau. After another day's travel, the second camel transfers one day's water to your camel, keeping two days' water to get back to Fort Beau. Meanwhile your camel still has four days' water left, enabling you to reach Fort Geste and deliver the vital message.

## CHAPTER 13

## 1 ONE WORD FITS ALL

**A** Book
**B** Quick
**C** Paper
**D** Fruit
**E** Search

# Useful websites

## GENERAL INFORMATION ON MEMORY

www.dana.org

www.gloo.com.au

www.memorise.org

www.memory-loss.org

www.newscientist.com/topic/brain
For more information and the latest research into how the brain works

www.pbs.org/wnet/brain/

www.sharpbrains.com

www.youramazingbrain.org/yourmemory/

## MEMORY TECHNIQUES

www.buildyourmemory.com

www.buzanworld.com

www.changingminds.org/techniques/memory/peg

www.mindtools.com

www.worldmemorychampionships.com

www.youramazingbrain.org/yourmemory

## MORE PUZZLES

### Creativity
www.cul.co.uk/creative/puzzles.htm

www.learning-tree.org.uk

### Long-term memory

www.lumosity.com

www.memoryjoggingpuzzles.com

### Memory and creativity

www.cul.co.uk/creative/puzzles.htm

www.enchantedmind.com/html/science/creative_memory.html

www.supplementsformemorytips.com/Improve-Memory-When-You-Improve-Creativity.html

### Memory and organization

www.npmanagement.org/Article_List/Articles/Organizational_Memory.htm

www.web-us.com/memory/improving_memory.htm

### Numerical reasoning

www.cut-the-knot.com

www.jimloy.com
For numerical riddles

www.krazydad.com
For Kakuro puzzles

www.riddles.com
For creative conundrums

www.visualmathlearning.com

### Remembering names and faces

www.howtoimprovememory.org/names-faces/

www.memory-key.com/improving/strategies/everyday/remembering-names-faces

www.mymemoryfix.com/remember_faces.html

### Remembering numbers

www.braingle.com/mind/test_numbers.php

www.memorise.org/lesson3.htm

### Short-term memory

www.everydayhealth.com/longevity/mental-fitness/brain-exercises-for-memory.aspx

www.free-sudoku-puzzles.com/games/memory-game/short-term-memory-game.php

www.fupa.com/play/Puzzles-free-games/short-term-memory

www.onlinegamescastle.com/game/short-term-memory

www2.stetson.edu/~efriedma/puzzle
For a huge range of puzzles

### Verbal reasoning

www.puzzlechoice.com
For crosswords, word searches, and word play games

www.wordplays.com
For more verbal games

### Visual reasoning and spatial awareness

www.mycoted.com

www.sharpbrains.com

# Index

**A**

acronym technique 47
acrostic technique 48–9
  mnemonics 100
  PIN recall 90
advert recall 61
aide mémoires 76
algebra 128–9
alphabet
  direction 156
  order 133
  peg system 50–1
  sequencing 151
alternative uses test 173
anagrams 139
analogy reasoning 156
angles 126
animals, recalling 14
anniversaries, recalling 79
antonyms 135
areas and volumes 127, 143
arithmetic *see* maths phobia
association triggers 26–7, 34–6, 39, 40–1, 56
averages 124

**B**

background information to help recall 101
bar sign recall 16
base grouping 117
base system for passwords 86–8
bat information 102
battles, body peg system for recall 105
beach items, acrostic technique 48
biographical memory 8, 72
birds, recalling 14
birthdays, recalling 75, 78
body peg system 105
book lists 63
bullet point information for revision 102

**C**

calculator challenge 123
calendar peg system 76–9
car parking recall 63
cast list method 75
chess
  moves 148
  position recall 21
childhood memories 73
Christmas present list acrostic 49
chunking 22–3, 52, 55
class recall 64
clock peg system 66–9
coding
  letters with letters 164–5
  morse code 166
  numbers and letters 156
  for passwords 85–6
cognition 9
  definition 8
collective nouns recall 107
colour, recall 16, 18, 20
compass system 54
conceptualization 172
consonant swap for passwords 88
context studying 20, 24, 39
creative power boosting 170–1
creativity 9
cyphers 164

**D**

days of the week peg system 64–5, 68–9
decimals 114
declarative memory 8
design creativity 174
diary dates 64, 65, 66–7, 76–9
  for passwords 85
dinner food recall 61
  restaurant meals 74
dinner party genius 30–41
directions recall 54–5
distraction

background noise 24
new information 25, 34–5, 37–9, 40–1, 46, 53, 67, 76, 106–7
Stroop Test 137
task recall 49
doodling 173
drinks orders, remembering 27

**E**

emotional associations 26
emotional intelligence 9
encoding 8
episodic memory 8
event dates recall 68–9, 75, 77, 78, 79
  life events 73, 74
explicit memory 8

**F**

faces, recall 26, 30–41
  association triggers 34–7, 39
  features 36–7
  funny faces 31
  job match and 34
  long-term memory 75
  pairing couples 38
  positional recall 32–3
  rating 30
  sequencing 34
  unfunny faces 31
family history 73
fractions 113–14
frequency analysis 165

**G**

general knowledge quiz 99, 101
geometry 126
graphs 112, 128–9
grouping objects 15

**H**

history recall 106
holidays
  acrostic technique for item recall 48

alphabet peg system for item recall 51
events recall 69
sensory memories 74
household chores recall
link system 47
rhyming number peg system 52

**I**
interference with recall *see* distraction
interviews
remembering dates 65
remembering names 35

**J**
jeopardy game 176
job match and face recall 34
joke punchline test 176
journeys
direction recall 54–5, 64
long-term memories 75
peg system 62, 63, 106

**K**
key finder 56–7
keyboard coding for passwords 86
Kim's game 22–3
knot tying recall 80

**L**
landmark recall 18, 147
Leetspeak 85
letters
coding 156, 164–5
counting puzzle 136
cyphers 164
frequency analysis 165
logical aptitude 161
for PIN recall 92
scrabble puzzle 136
substitution puzzle 164
linguistic aptitude *see* verbal aptitude
link system 46
linking knowledge quiz 99
list recall 22, 23, 63
logical aptitude 9, 154–67

rating 154
long-term memory 8, 72–81
boosting mundane recall 44–59
rating 72

**M**
map reading 18, 19, 147
maths phobia 9, 110–19, 122–9
arithmetic test 111
rating 122
*see also* numbers
medication mnemonic 67
medium-term memory 8, 60–81
rating 60
memorization for revision practice 104
memory 8–9
biographical 8
declarative 8
definition 8
episodic 8
long-term *see* long-term memory
medium-term *see* medium-term
memory
procedural 8
short-term *see* short-term memory
working 8
memory house system 45
mental arithmetic 119
mental mapping 103
mental rotation 144–7
mind web technique 103
mnemonics
acrostic technique 100
for medications 67
for PIN recall 93
money test 111–12, 116, 118
morse code 166
multi-store model 8
multitasking *see* distraction
musical instruments, body peg system
for recall 105

**N**
names recall 30–41
for passwords 85

narrative peg system 106
nominative determinism 34
numbers
coding with letters 156
interference with recall 25
missing, working out 118
PIN recall 90–5
practicing mental arithmetic 119
prime 123
puzzles 123, 124–6
recall 14
*see also* maths phobia; rhyming
number peg system
numerical aptitude 9, 110–19
rating 110
nursery rhymes for PIN recall 94

**O**
objects
alternative uses test 173
categorizing 171
fantastical creativity 175
listing 22, 23
locating and grouping 15, 19
pairing 22, 23
random object recall 13
odd one out puzzle 136
operas, journey peg system for recall
106
order recall 34
origami 81

**P**
pairing faces 38
pairing objects 22, 23
paper folding recall 81
password recall 84–9, 91, 95
peg system
alphabet 50–1
body 105
calendar 76–9
clock 66–9
days of the week 64–5, 68–9
journey 62–3, 106
narrative stages 106

rhyming number 52, 78, 79
percentages 115–16, 119
pictures in mind's eye, recall 17
PIN recall 84, 90–5
poets, recalling 107
positional recall 15, 19, 21, 32–3
prime numbers 123
problem solving 176
procedural memory 8, 72, 80
prompts for passwords 85
proportions 115

Q

quizzes 99

R

random object recall 13, 15
reading upside down 137
reasoning see logical aptitude
recall 8
   triggers 26
remote associates test 171
repetition for recall 21, 31
revision practice 102–7
rhyming number peg system 52, 78, 79
   for PIN recall 94

S

semantic memory 72, 76, 98–107
   rating 98
sensory memories 74
sequencing
   alphabet 151
   faces 34
   materials 155
   shape 149–51, 155
   words 157, 161
shape
   fitting 148
   recall 13, 38
   rotation 144–7
   sequencing 149–51, 155
shopping
   acronym technique 47
   acrostic technique 48, 49

alphabet peg system 50
chunking 53
linking system 45–7
list recall 45
money test 111–12
rhyming number peg system 52
short-term memory 8, 12–29
   boosting mundane recall 44–59
   decay 21, 24
   later recall 24
   rating 12, 44
sightseeing items recall 51
sleepover items acrostic 48
social intelligence see emotional
   intelligence
spatial distance for problem solving 176
spot the difference puzzle 143
story creativity 175, 176
Stroop Test 137
symbols for passwords 85
synonyms 134

T

task recall
   acrostic technique 47, 49
   alphabet peg system 50
   journey peg system 62
   rhyming number peg system 52
telephone callers, recall 61
temporal distance for problem solving
   176
three-step booster 40–1
tile game 148
time logic puzzle 155
timing test 117
traffic sign recall 17
triggers for STM recall 26
true or false questions 160
TV programme recall 68

V

Venn diagrams 158–9
verbal aptitude 9
   rating 132
visualization triggers

diary dates 64–7, 76–9
directions 54
faces 26–7, 39, 40–1, 75
journeys 62
key finder 57
PIN recall 93
revision practice 103, 104–5
visuo-spatial aptitude 9, 142–51
volumes and areas 127

W

waypoints 55
weekday peg system see days of the
   week peg system
weights and measures 118
words
   grid puzzles 136
   opposites conceptualization 172
   for PIN number recall 91, 93
   reading upside down 137
   remote associates test 171
   sequencing 157, 161
   verbal aptitude 132–9
   word ladders 138
   within words 138
writing, creative 175–6

# About the author

**Joel Levy** is a science writer and journalist with special interest in psychology. His writing explores both mainstream and fringe psychology, from cognitive boosting to anomalous experiences. After taking degrees in molecular biology and psychology at Warwick and Edinburgh universities, he has gone on to write books including *Boost Your IQ* and *Train Your Brain*.

# About the illustrator

**Keith Hagan's** richly varied career in the graphic arts spans the disciplines of illustration, film special effects animation, graphic design and art direction, and commercial copywriting. He continues to create visual and written material for publishing, advertising, and corporate clients.

# Author's acknowledgments

Thanks to Lizzie Yeates and the rest of the team behind the book: Angela Baynham, Miranda Harvey, Harriet Yeomans and Keith Hagan. Special thanks also to Dawn Henderson. Personal dedication to Anne Hooper, an inspiration and heroic source of support.

# Publisher's acknowledgments

Dorling Kindersley would like to thank Kate Fenton and Heather Matthews for design assistance, Michele Clarke for supplying the index, Claire Cross for proofreading, Nikki Sims for checking the puzzles and exercises, and to Roger Trevena for checking the puzzles in the two mathematical chapters.